FRAMEWORKS

DAMS and

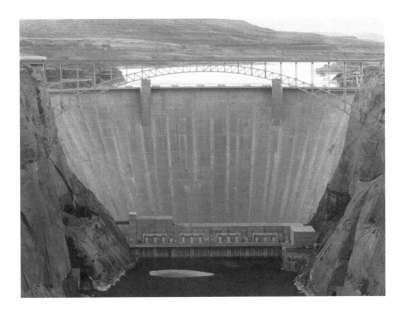

WATERWAYS

Shana Priwer

Cynthia Phillips

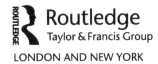

Routledge
Taylor & Francis Group

LONDON AND NEW YORK

First published 2009 by M.E. Sharpe

Published 2015 by Routledge
2 Park Square, Milton Park, Abingdon, Oxon OX14 4RN
711 Third Avenue, New York, NY 10017, USA

Routledge is an imprint of the Taylor & Francis Group, an informa business

Library of Congress Cataloging-in-Publication Data

Phillips, Cynthia.
  Dams and waterways / Cynthia Phillips and Shana Priwer.
    p. cm. -- (Frameworks)
  Includes bibliographical references and index.
  ISBN 978-0-7656-8122-5 (hardcover : alk. paper)
  1. Dams—Juvenile literature. 2. Waterways—Juvenile literature. 3. Hydraulic engineering—Juvenile literature. 4. Water-power—Juvenile literature. 5. Irrigation—Juvenile literature. I. Priwer, Shana. II. Title.

TC540.P45 2008
627--dc22

                    2007040699

ISBN 13: 9780765681225 (hpk)

Editor: Peter Mavrikis
Production Manager: Henrietta Toth
Editorial Assistant and Photo Research: Alison Morretta
Program Coordinator: Cathy Prisco
Design: Patrice Sheridan
Line Art: FoxBytes

PICTURE CREDITS: Front cover: Gallo Images/Getty Images; title page: Dorling Kindersley/Getty Images; pages 6, 11, 42, 60, 62: Time & Life Pictures/Getty Images; pages 8 (left), 8 (right), 10, 21 (top), 21 (bottom), 26 (bottom), 30, 38 (left), 38 (right), 39 (left), 39 (right), 41, 52, 53, 54, 56, 98 (bottom), 100: FoxBytes; page 13: Nordic Photos/Getty Images; page 17: Visuals Unlimited/Getty Images; pages 18, 23, 36: National Geographic/Getty Images; pages 24, 31, 73: Science Faction/Getty Images; page 25: China Photos/Getty Images; pages 26 (top), 40, 61, 95, 104: Stone/Getty Images; pages 32, 55: Dorling Kindersley/Getty Images; pages 34, 45, 57: Photographer's Choice/Getty Images; pages 35, 81, 92, 96, 98 (top), 103: Getty Images; pages 43, 69: China Span/Getty Images; pages 47, 76, 84, 101: Associated Press; page 48: Sebun Photo/Getty Images; page 50: Discovery Channel Images/Getty Images; page 64: Gallo Images/Getty Images; page 65: Photonica/Getty Images; page 67: De Agostini Picture Library/Getty Images; page 70: Library of Congress; pages 78, 94: AFP/Getty Images; page 80: Alinari/Art Resource, NY; pages 88 (top), 88 (middle), 88 (bottom): NOAA/Getty Images; back cover: Photographer's Choice/Getty Images.

CONTENTS

ABOUT

FRAMEWORKS

Architecture has undergone sweeping development since people first constructed shelter. In ancient cultures, most architecture was temporary because it accommodated nomadic populations. As communities began to grow roots, so did their architecture. Whether they were residential, commercial, religious, or civic, structures of permanence slowly appeared on the global landscape.

Over time, specific aesthetics and structural techniques developed. Advancements in the physical sciences allowed engineers to create increasingly complex works. Temples became more elaborate, buildings grew ever taller, and bridges spanned bodies of water that only boats had dared to cross before. Once science and design crossed paths, there was no turning back.

The goal of the FRAMEWORKS series is to provide insight into the science behind the structures that are part of our everyday lives, from the skills developed by the Egyptians in building pyramids to the application of advanced hydroelectric technology in modern-day dams. Basic concepts in mathematics, physics, and engineering help illustrate the science that supports the creation of increasingly complex structures.

This series assumes no prior knowledge of advanced math and physics but, rather, builds the reader's understanding by explaining scientific concepts in common terms, as well as with simple equations. Engaging examples illustrate ideas such as mass, force, speed, and energy. Case studies from real-world projects demonstrate the application of these concepts. Stories of famous structural disasters serve an important purpose in showing how, even for professional architects and engineers, gaining knowledge is an ongoing process.

DAMS AND WATERWAYS covers the range of ways in which water has been used, corralled, manipulated, harnessed, and otherwise turned into far more than a basic requirement for life. Transportation, building, manufacturing, and energy production are just a few examples of major businesses that have historically relied on water to increase efficiency.

Irrigation, or supplying water to crops and farmland, has long been recognized as necessary to grow enough food to meet the needs of a growing population. Canals and aqueducts have been used for thousands of years to aid farmers in this endeavor. The distribution of drinking water is a cultural and societal task that is in everyone's best interest; water towers and water-pumping windmills aid the public water distribution system. Putting water to work through the use of waterwheels was a life-altering invention that helped to spark a boom in industrialization in many regions around the world.

Dams are another way in which the power of water has been harnessed. While the purpose of early dams was mainly to retain water for drinking and irrigation, massive modern dams are also used to generate hydroelectric power. Turbine engines aid in the generation of a form of power that is both clean and renewable. While large dams have ecological consequences of their own, some are capable of generating enough power to sustain entire regions.

It was hard to beat water for transporting large amounts of goods in the time before air travel. Man-made transportation canals came into heavy usage and greatly facilitated settlement and trade. Canals were designed using the best engineering knowledge available at the time, and most were quite successful. There are several examples, however, in which miscalculations in the design of dams and canals have resulted in horrific consequences.

Water has tremendous power to aid and support human life, and yet that same power can become destructive as a result of nature as well as human error. Dikes, seawalls, and flood barriers are all structures that serve mainly to protect citizens from water gone awry. They vary in their construction and efficiency, and unfortunately each can result in environmental fallout. Managing water successfully is very much a balancing act between meeting human needs and preserving as much as possible of the natural environment.

The FRAMEWORKS series provides an entertaining and educational approach to the science of building. Read on to learn about the ways in which science supports, literally, our built environment.

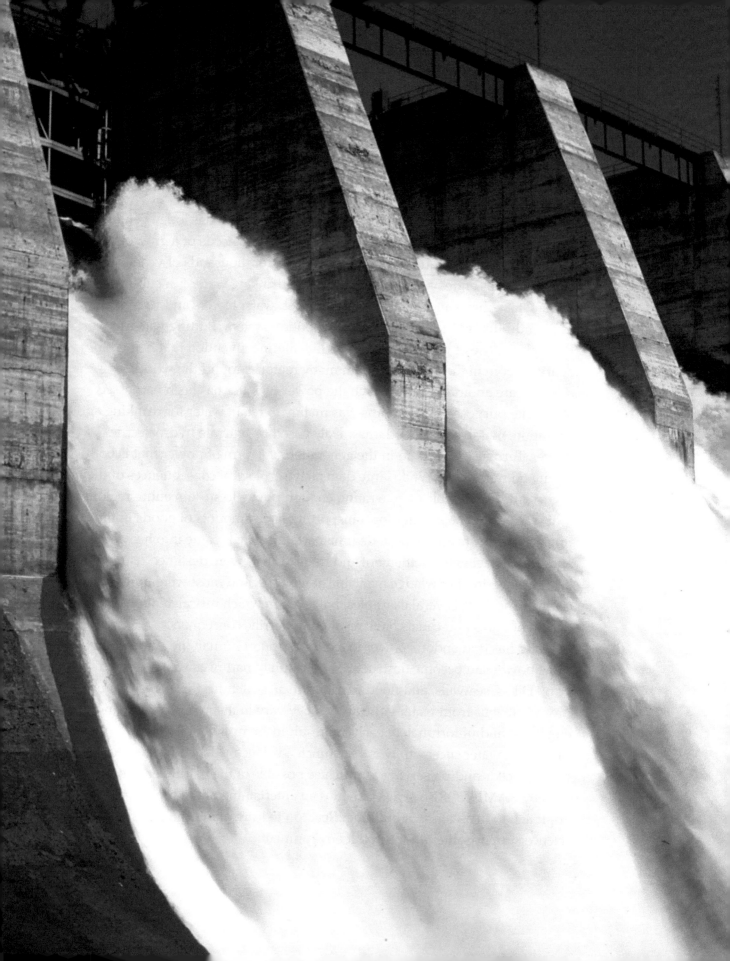

1

THE BASICS OF WATER SUPPLY

The Canadian Shipshaw Dam generates a substantial amount of hydroelectric power and was built to power the Canadian aluminum industry.

Seventy-one percent of our planet is covered with water, and water is essential to all life on Earth. Water makes up about 60 percent of the human body, which requires at least a half-gallon (2 liters) of water each day to survive. In addition to drinking water, people need water for irrigating crops and transporting people and goods. Human settlements have always centered around sources of water, from desert oases to bustling seaports.

Water is also an important power source. In the early days of industry, water powered mills that sawed lumber and produced cloth. Today, water is used to generate electricity in huge hydroelectric plants where dams have been built across some of the largest rivers in the world.

PROPERTIES OF WATER

Why is water so special? In its most basic form, water is a common liquid with no color or smell. However, water has specific chemical and physical properties that make it different from most other substances on Earth.

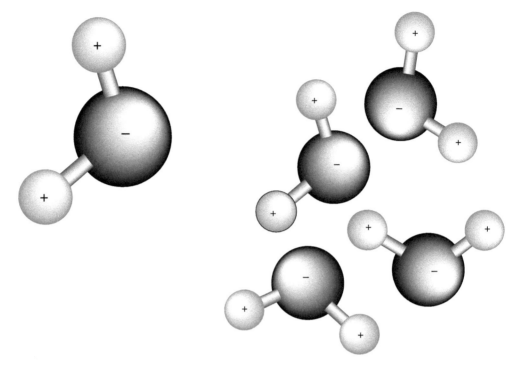

First is its molecular structure. Water has a very simple chemical formula: one water molecule is made up of two hydrogen atoms that are bound to one oxygen atom. The chemical formula for water is H_2O.

Due to the properties of the oxygen atom, the two hydrogen atoms stick to a single side of the oxygen atom, rather than one on each side. The water molecule is therefore not symmetric, and becomes like a magnet: the side with the hydrogen atoms ends up with a negative charge, and the other side has a positive charge.

This chemical structure allows water molecules to stick to one another. The negative side of one water molecule attracts the positive side of another water molecule and this attraction results in clumps of water. This "stickiness" yields high surface tension (the attractive force of molecules on water's surface), which causes water to hold together in drops.

While most materials can be found only as a solid, a liquid, or a gas at the surface of the Earth, water can exist in all three phases. Water's three forms are solid ice, liquid water, and gaseous steam.

Water's physical properties cause it to form a crystal structure when it freezes, and it is one of the only substances on Earth that is actually less dense in a solid state (ice) than it is in a liquid state (water). This varied density explains why ice floats in water. With most other substances the solid form sinks to the bottom of the liquid. For example, if salt crystals form out of a salt solution, the crystals will fall to the bottom of the container rather than float on top.

Water is also sometimes called the "universal solvent" because many substances can be dissolved in it.

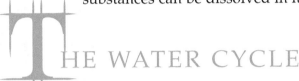

THE WATER CYCLE

Water is always in motion. The water cycle describes the movement of water from solid to liquid to gas and the physical movement of water over the surface of the earth. Starting in the clouds, which are made up of tiny drops of water vapor, water eventually reaches a high enough concentration to precipitate out as rain. Under the right conditions, raindrops may freeze into delicate crystalline snowflakes and land on mountaintops or in cold regions. There, water is stored in the form of snow. When summer comes, the snow melts and liquid water runs down from the mountains in streams and rivers or in underground aquifers.

From the potential energy of an ice pack at the top of a mountain, liquid water converts into kinetic energy as it travels downhill. Potential energy is stored energy, and kinetic energy is the energy that results from the motion of a body. The flowing water may eventually reach a large pond or lake, or it may travel all the way to the ocean. Since water is a liquid, it forms an equipotential surface. This means that sea level is approximately the same absolute distance from the center of the earth everywhere on the globe (except for variations due to temperature, pressure, and other factors). Reaching an equipotential surface halts the downward motion of water, which stops when it reaches a stable lake or ocean that is at sea level or has no outlets for water to continue its downward journey. Heat energy is transferred to the water by sunlight, which eventually causes some of the water to evaporate. This water vapor ascends into the atmosphere, where it forms clouds and eventually rain, and the water cycle begins again.

This diagram of the water cycle shows how water is stored in the natural environment as ice, snow, and ground water; events such as runoff, evaporation, and condensation complete the circular nature of water's motion from atmosphere to land to ocean and back to atmosphere.

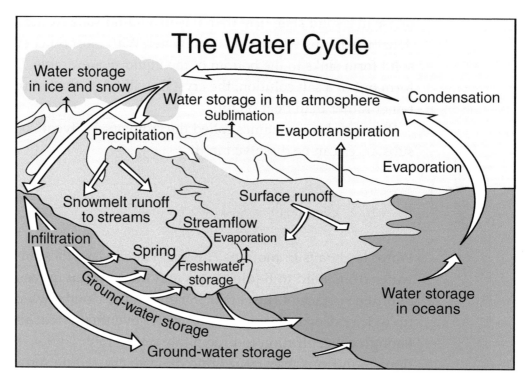

WATER AND EARLY AGRICULTURE

Early humans were primarily hunters and gatherers who moved around the countryside, traveling to where plants and animals were abundant in different seasons. Eventually they understood that if they planted crops and domesticated animals, they could create a stable food source rather than following game and vegetation as the seasons changed. As more stable societies were formed, the development of agriculture allowed larger groups of people to remain in one place all year round.

Irrigation is an important element of any agricultural society. Forests and grasslands tend to grow naturally and flourish and wither with the seasons. But humans rely on plants for food and cannot be at the mercy of nature. In most areas of the world, but particularly in those that have long hot summers, plants must be watered if they are going to survive and produce food. Early farmers probably planted crops in areas that were naturally wet and lush. As civilizations expanded, the land available for farming was more marginal and often required additional water to be fully productive.

Early irrigation was likely as simple as carrying a bucket or other container of water from a river or spring to where crops were grown. Major agricultural areas required more substantial irrigation to support growing populations. The area of the world located in the Middle East and northern Africa along the Nile, Tigris, Euphrates, and Indus rivers is often called the cradle of civilization because of the early cities that were located there. In regions like Egypt, the only fertile land was near a river. Early settlers could easily increase the amount of arable land by building dams and canals to store and transport water to drier outlying areas.

Farmers along major rivers also took advantage of natural cycles to help support their crops. In the Nile River valley, for example, the river goes through a flood stage approximately once a year. During this period, water flow increases, and sediment transport rises dramatically. The

Traditional irrigation can consist of human-powered watering, seen here as a woman carries water directly to the fields.

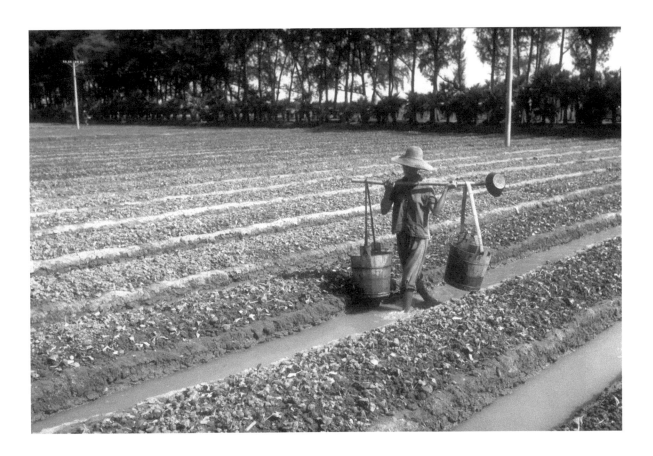

LIFE IN THE TROPICS

In tropical parts of the world such as Belize, Bali, and Cambodia, early civilizations were spread out rather than being concentrated around major rivers. Tropical parts of the world have large seasonal variations in rainfall, which produce wet and dry seasons rather than the familiar hot and cold seasons experienced in more temperate parts of the world. One of the main issues for people living in tropical regions is water storage during the dry season. Some early tropical civilizations, such as the Maya, built reservoirs on hilltops to capture rainwater from the wet season and save it for use during the dry season. These reservoirs and other ways of saving water for the dry months produced a tropical concentration of civilizations that was decentralized, resulting in more small settlements and fewer large cities than found in semi-arid regions that depended on rivers.

faster flow and higher volume of water during the flooding stage causes dirt and organic material to be picked up by the river and deposited high on the banks of the river.

While river floods can be disastrous for permanent cities built near rivers, in ancient times they were recognized as a beneficial part of a river's cycle. The flood stage deposited fresh, rich dirt full of nutrients. This richer soil helped nourish the next season's crops as a kind of natural fertilizer. In Egypt, this annual flood was called the gift of the Nile.

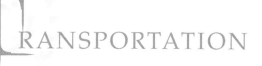

TRANSPORTATION

As civilizations grew in complexity, the way they used water began to change. The transportation goods rapidly grew in importance as trade increased and became more specialized. Spices from Asia could be traded for furs from North America, for example, or for gold jewelry from South America.

Raw materials such as lumber also had to be transported. Early traders had only two methods of transport available: over land on animals or over water on boats. Boats can carry larger loads and travel much faster than pack animals, so transporting goods on water is more efficient even if the actual distance traveled is longer. For instance, in the eighteenth

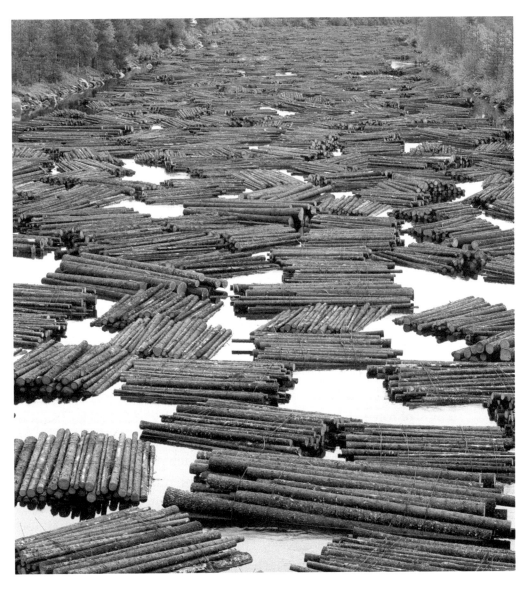

One of the most cost-effective means of transporting lumber is to float it downstream. Logs are tied together in batches and are guided along their path as necessary.

13

and nineteenth centuries in the United States, before the Panama Canal and the intercontinental railroad were built, it was often cheaper and faster to send something by boat all the way down around the southern tip of South America than it was to send it by land from the East Coast to the West Coast!

Transportation of goods and passengers by water was a huge industry. Its economic importance was a major reason that large cities often developed in favorable ports, such as New York and San Francisco. Many port cities were also established on major rivers. Raw materials such as lumber could easily be floated down rivers on barges to sawmills and other industrial destinations.

Even today, although airplanes can travel around the globe in a matter of hours, it is very expensive for companies to send large quantities of raw materials and finished products by air. Large, heavy loads are transported across the oceans on giant ships that carry huge metal containers filled with various products. The goods are unloaded at ports and then travel inland on tractor-trailer trucks or freight trains. A single ship can hold hundreds of containers, while a truck usually carries only one or two. For raw materials and goods that can make the month-long trip across the ocean, water is still the transportation method of choice.

In addition to using naturally available bodies of water for transportation, engineers have designed canals to connect bodies of water. The earliest canals probably grew from irrigation channels, which were widened to allow passage of shallow-bottomed boats or barges. There are several advantages to traveling over water rather than land. First, properly designed boats are buoyant, which means that the water supports the weight of the object being transported. This makes even very large, heavy objects, such as tree trunks, relatively easy to maneuver with a minimum of force. Second, transporting goods by water rather than over land reduces overall friction, which is the loss of energy due to heat dissipation. A wheeled cart dissipates much more energy through friction than a boat in water, and so the boat is the more efficient means of transportation. Third, because water is an equipotential surface, the surface of a canal or river is always flat (with the exception of small local disturbances such as waves). This makes travel much easier and smoother than traversing a bumpy or hilly road, or a mountain. In addition, water will always travel in a downhill direction, and boats traveling downstream can take advantage of the natural current of a river to further reduce the required energy expended to transport materials. Lumber is often transported from forests to sawmills in as simple a fashion as possible: large, rough-hewn logs are simply tied together to form rafts that are then floated downstream. Imagine trying to transport a single large log, let alone dozens, over land with such a small expenditure of energy!

Water has incredible value to society. In addition to the all-important task of keeping humans and food sources alive, water helps to harness energy and ease the transportation of goods.

MEANDERING RIVERS

The shortest distance between two points may be a straight line, but rivers do not always follow that rule. In fact, though rivers in general travel from higher ground to lower regions, they tend to curve along their path. The reason for this behavior is that as a river moves around a small curve, the water tends to move faster around the outside of a bend and more slowly around the inside of a bend. This pattern of motion allows the water to move together as a unit—the distance along the outside of a curve is longer than along the inside of a curve, so just like members of a marching band in a parade going around a bend, the water outside must move faster to keep up with the rest of the river.

Water that moves faster cannot carry as much sediment. Rivers generally erode material from the outside of the curve, where the water is moving faster, and deposit the material they are carrying on the inside of the curve, where the water is moving more slowly. Over time, the curves get larger and larger until they actually form a circle. The river then follows the straight-line rule and breaks through to continue downstream. The rest of the curve can be cut off from the river, forming a lake called an "oxbow" lake because it is shaped like a kind of harness that was once used on oxen.

These river curves are called meanders, named by the ancient Greeks after a particularly curving river called the Meander River in what is now Turkey. Over time, the meanders change in size and location as the river constantly makes small changes in its course, dropping sand and rocks in one place and eroding them from the banks in another. While this is the natural course of rivers, city planners prefer that their rivers stay in one place; planning for roads and bridges can be very difficult if a river changes course. Farmers and homeowners also depend on being a certain distance from a river. It could be devastating for a farmer if the water source suddenly moved out of irrigation range, while a homeowner would prefer that his house not suddenly be chosen as the site for a new meander.

In some urban environments the riverbanks are cemented in, forcing the river to stay in one location. Preventing the river from moving naturally, however, has consequences. The river tends to move more quickly when it is forced into a straight, clean pathway, meaning that erosion can increase both upstream and downstream of the cemented portion of the river's path. In addition, as a natural river changes course, it mixes up the soil of the whole river valley. The end result is fertile soil for agriculture that will be lost if the river can no longer meander.

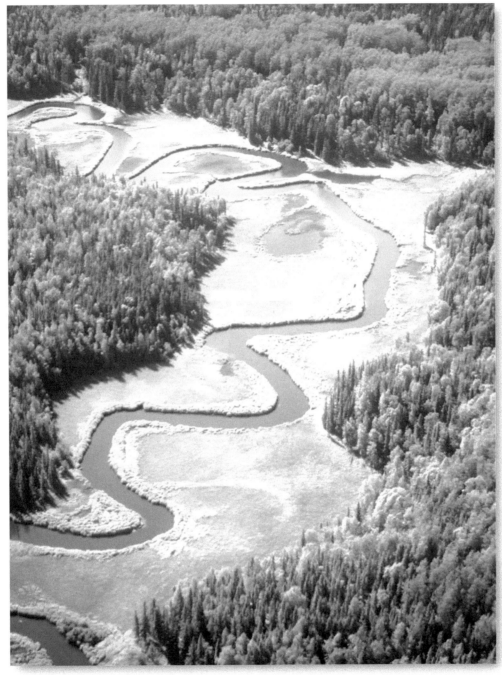

A meandering river in Alaska, with an oxbow lake in the middle where the river has broken through a curve.

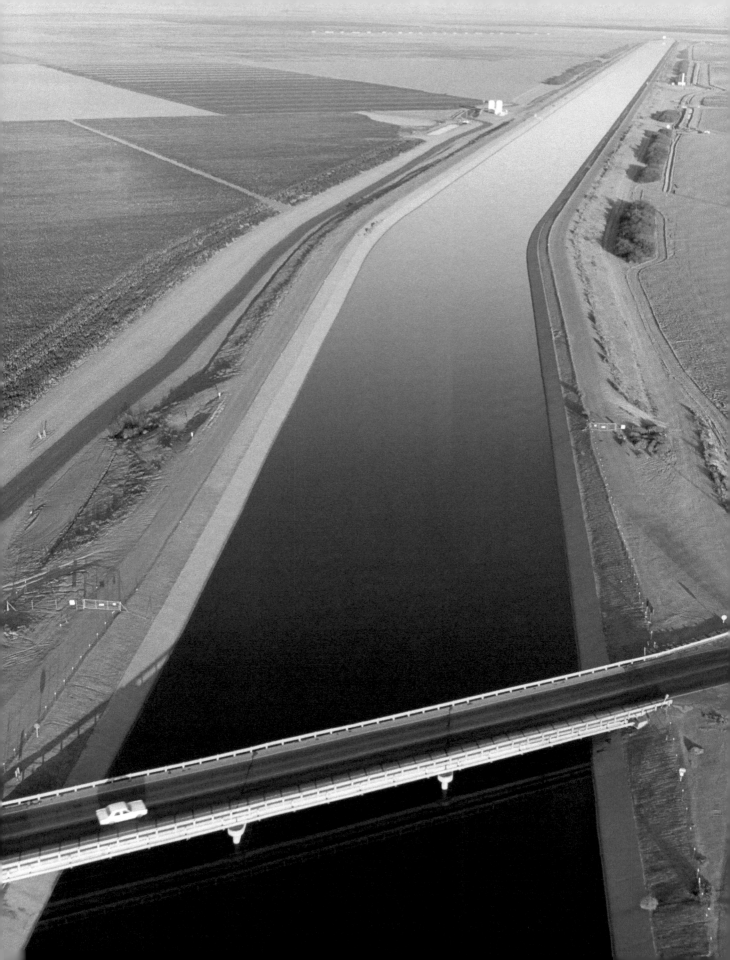

2

IRRIGATION AND DRINKING WATER

The California Aqueduct is about 400 miles (645 km) long, and serves to transport water from northern to southern California. It allows inhabitants of desert-like communities to survive where they might otherwise be forced to live closer to a water source.

Most people take it for granted that when a faucet is turned on, safe drinking water will come out. This is a modern convenience that most people would not be willing to live without, but indoor plumbing and the ability to run a hot bath, flush a toilet, or water a lawn are fairly recent developments.

Since the beginning of time, humans have sought and used water for drinking and cooking. While early nomadic cultures traveled around and remained close to water sources, people who later settled in more permanent civilizations had to devise methods of ensuring access to sufficient water to meet their needs. Over the years, ancient cultures developed different ways of transporting water to their towns and villages. As time went on, these methods became more and more advanced, culminating in the modern water delivery system in place throughout most developed countries today.

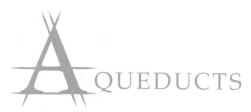

AQUEDUCTS

Aqueducts are huge structures that transport water from one place to another. The ancient Egyptians and other early civilizations created aqueducts, but the best-preserved examples from ancient times were built by the Romans throughout the Roman Empire. Most of these aqueducts were built between 312 B.C.E. and 226 C.E.

The aqueducts throughout the Roman Empire were some of the longest and most permanent, and many of them survive today. The simplest Roman aqueducts consisted of a deep channel that was dug into the rocky countryside. A constant, small gradient was maintained to make sure that water always flowed downhill to the desired location. Because the water had to be consistently flowing, and the means for achieving this flow was primarily gravity, these "natural" aqueducts tended to meander along with the terrain and rarely ran in a straight line from place to place.

Over time, and as cities were built farther from water sources, there was an increased need for more formalized and sturdier water transport systems. In places where the natural terrain was not at the right level to allow the gradual downhill gradient needed to sustain flow, artificial supports were built. Aqueducts built within arched structures, which provided a tall and stable structural form, were typical in Roman architecture. Sometimes channels were built on top of stone walls. This technique was less expensive and faster to construct than a full arch.

Multiple vertical layers of arches were sometimes used to gain height for the aqueduct to cross a deep valley and maintain flow on either side. At the very top of these immense stone aqueducts was a simple channel through which the water flowed. Gradually, larger and taller arched structures were built to allow water to travel even longer distances and across valleys or other gaps in the landscape. Some early aqueducts traveled as far as 50 miles (80 kilometers) or more!

Underground Flow

The majority of actual water transport took place in underground trenches. In a time when warfare and marauding enemies were common, the

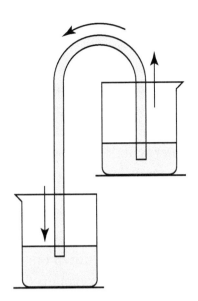

A siphon takes advantage of hydrostatic pressure to move liquids from a high destination to a second, lower destination. Pumping is not required, but a change in elevation from source to destination is necessary.

water supply was safer if kept underground. Pipes were also used as the terrain required.

Sediment tanks were built along the aqueduct route to capture debris. Cisterns were eventually added to the aqueduct system. These tanks stored water that could later be pumped out. Cisterns were sometimes large arched structures that were eventually connected to a system of underground pipes for distribution. Another advantage of elevated cisterns was that water could be pumped into the city at a higher pressure.

In most closed aqueducts, ventilation holes were drilled to ensure that the water moving into the city was fresh and that excess air pressure did not build up inside the channels. But how could water be encouraged to leap across a valley that was too large for the architectural requirements of the aqueduct or in a place where building an aqueduct across the valley would have been too expensive? The solution of the day, which still finds use in modern times, was to create a closed channel that went down into the valley and back up the other side. This channel was later called an inverted siphon, or a continuous pipe that allowed water across different elevations.

Inverted siphons use a U-shaped tunnel to channel liquids from one place to another. A common example of an inverted siphon is the trap under the kitchen sink.

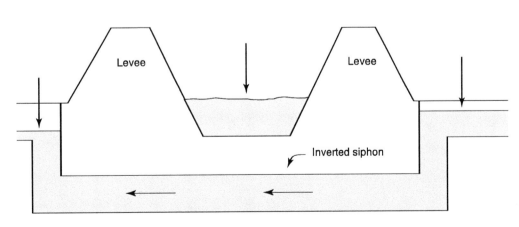

A siphon is a system that allows a liquid from an upper reservoir to travel through a tube or pipe to a lower reservoir. In a traditional siphon, as long as the lower end of the tube is located below the bottom of the upper reservoir, the middle of the tube can rise higher than the top water level, and the water will continue to flow. For example, if a tube is placed in a large bucket of water and travels up over the side and then down below the bottom of the bucket, water will flow through the tube and over the side even though it must initially travel uphill to do so. The behavior of siphons is governed by Bernoulli's equation, which helps predict how high the intermediate point in the siphon can be for various liquids.

An inverted siphon is a simple device. It is a closed tube or pipe through which water can flow. Water can flow down one side of a valley in this U-shaped pipe and then flow uphill to travel up the other side. The water in its initial position at the top of the hill has gravitational

BERNOULLI

The mathematician Daniel Bernoulli was born in Holland but spent much of his life in Switzerland, where he was a professor at the University of Basel. He studied various areas of math and theoretical physics, and his biggest contribution was what is known as Bernoulli's equation. This equation is a fundamental part of fluid mechanics and helps describe why airplanes can fly.

Bernoulli's equation states that if the velocity of a fluid increases, then the pressure must decrease at the same time, or the energy of position of the fluid due to gravity must change. Like most physics theories, this exact description only applies to a certain type of idealized fluid, with no external work being done on the system. Bernoulli's equation comes directly from the application of the principle of conservation of energy to a fluid system. In addition to airplane flight calculations, the principle can also be applied to how siphons work.

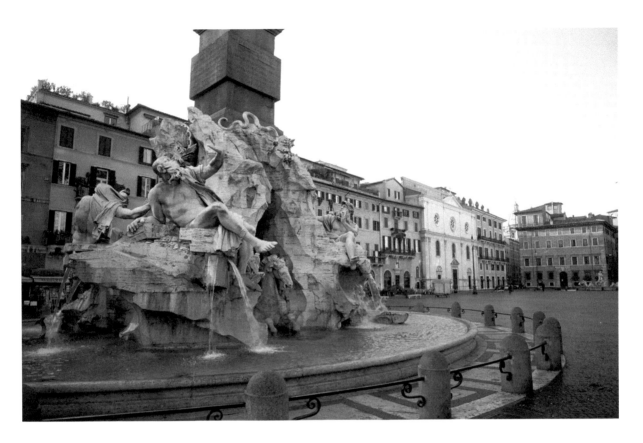

The gravity-fed fountain at the Roman Piazza del Popolo contains sculptures depicting scenes from Roman mythology. The fountain is only one component of this piazza, which serves as a communal gathering point and celebration of Roman history.

potential energy, which is transformed into kinetic energy as the water travels down the pipe to the bottom of the valley. That kinetic energy, coupled with the pressure exerted on the water by the water above it in the pipe, allows it to travel back up the other side of the valley to approximately the same height.

Public fountains in ancient Rome were beautiful as well as functional. Although some of Rome's larger buildings (especially those for royalty) had fresh water pumped directly in, most people had to walk to a public fountain, fill buckets with fresh water, and carry them home. Because of the water pressure that resulted from storing the water in a high cistern, fountains were also capable of spraying water out into the pools below.

Aqueducts are still in use today. The state of California has three major aqueducts that bring water into southern California from northern California and from the Colorado River. Aqueducts are used in countries throughout the world for supplying city dwellers with drinking water, as well as providing water for crop irrigation.

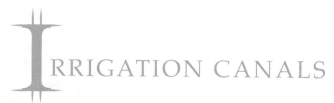

IRRIGATION CANALS

In places where farming is the main means of subsistence, getting water to the crops is a very important task. Thousands of years ago, a fairly simple mechanism was devised to accomplish this: the irrigation canal. This was a long, man-made ditch that diverted water from a nearby river or lake. The canal was angled slightly downward so that the force of gravity would cause the channel to fill up with water that was then diverted to fields and other locations where farmers needed easy access to a water supply.

One of the earliest major examples of an irrigation canal is the Nahrwan Canal, dating to about 2400 B.C.E. This canal, located in modern-day Iraq, was nearly 185 miles (300 kilometers) long. It supplied water for irrigation as well as for drinking and allowed civilizations to flourish in parts of the region that would otherwise have been unsustainable.

An effective means of irrigating fields is the use of drip irrigation. Canals channel water to central locations, and the water is distributed to the crops via drip tapes.

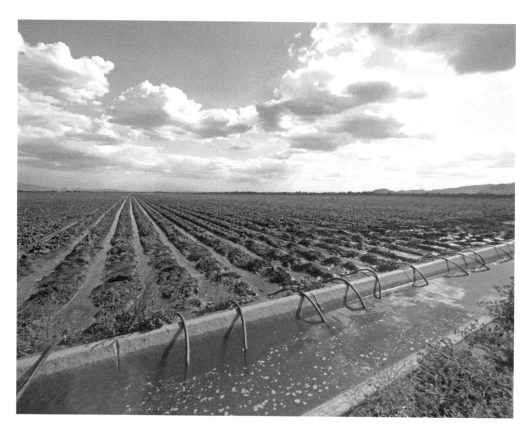

Another example of an early canal is the Grand Canal in China. Construction on this massive building project began around 485 B.C.E. and was completed around 610 C.E. The total length of this canal is 1,115 miles (1,795 kilometers) and is spanned by nearly sixty bridges. Twenty-four locks have been added over the years. A navigation lock is a chamber that allows boats to travel the canal in places where the water level changes, usually due to the surrounding terrain. Because the Grand Canal is so very large, it had more uses than as a typical irrigation canal. It was also the major route for the transportation of goods, such as grain and building supplies, between different parts of China.

Dujiangyan Dam and Irrigation System

One of the most sophisticated early canals was built in China around 256 B.C.E. The Dujiangyan dam and irrigation system was designed by Li Bing, a provincial governor. The system was designed not only as a dam to block flooding on the Minjiang River, but also to provide irrigation to nearby farmland and to support boat travel. Part of the river is split into an aque-

The Dujiangyan Water Conservancy Project in China is one of the world's oldest water structures, dating back to the third century B.C.E. Still in use today, it helps irrigate crops by providing water via gravity feed.

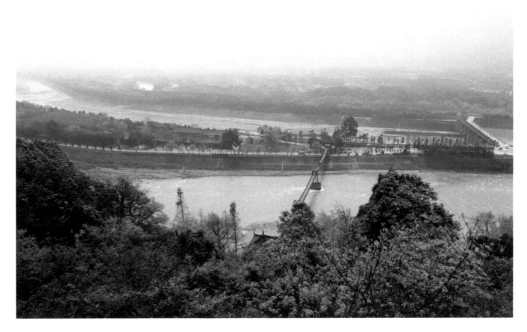

duct that leads to a nearby city, and a dike in the river keeps silt from traveling into the aqueduct and clogging it. The ancient designers of the irrigation system clearly understood that slowing the pace of the water would reduce its kinetic energy and reduce the amount of sediment it could transport.

The dike divides the river into inner and outer portions. The amount of water that is diverted into the aqueduct changes with the flow rates of different seasons. The spillway was originally constructed from bamboo cages that were filled with stones and piled on top of each other in the river to form a diversion channel. If the water-flow rate was too high, the water could simply flow over the tops of the cages (which now are built from concrete) and reach the rest of the river.

Building a structure of this size was quite difficult in the days before explosives were invented. The engineers managed to cut a channel through the mountains by intermittently applying heat and cold to the rocks. The cycling between two temperature extremes eventually weakened the rock, allowing it to be broken more easily and removed. Today—2,000 years later—the Dujiangyan system still provides the city of Chengdu with water.

WATER TOWERS

Water towers are a common marker of modern civilization. Many towns have several water towers scattered around. These large tanks of water are set up high in a tower. The average size for a water tower is around 50 feet (15 meters) in diameter, and they usually stand between 75 and 200 feet (22 and 60 meters) tall. Most are designed to hold about a one-day supply of water for the area that they serve, and they are generally located on the highest ground possible.

Water for any community has to come from a source, such as a river, lake, or reservoir. After being treated to remove bacteria and other undesirable contaminants, water is pumped into the local system's pipes. For residents of a city to receive water, some energy must be applied to the water in order to move it from the source to the desired location. That energy can be created using different methods, such as pumps or a gravity feed. Gravity feeds are only effective in areas where water flows from

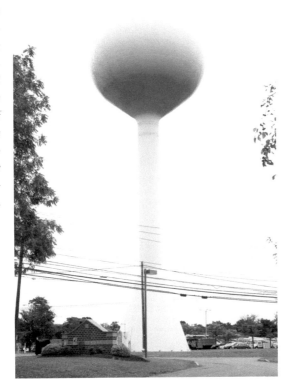

Water towers take on a characteristic look in the landscape, and often signify the presence of a community in what otherwise might be solely farmland.

high elevations to low ones, whereas pumps can be used regardless of the terrain. A water tower allows a gravity-feed system to be used even in a flat location.

A water tower is directly connected to local water pipes and maintains a constant level of pressure within the water system because of its elevation. Water is pumped into the tower during low-use hours and is then drained from the system during periods of high usage (such as when everyone runs their dishwashers in the evening). With the pressure advantage of the

Water towers work to raise the pressure of water in city pipes and help ensure that water is ready and waiting when people turn on their kitchen faucets in the morning.

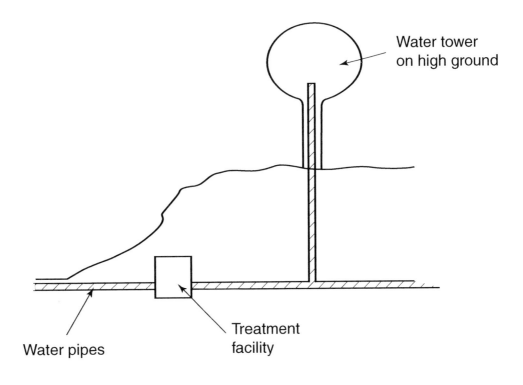

Water tower on high ground

Treatment facility

Water pipes

WATER TOWERS FOR TALL BUILDINGS

Most small towns have a water tower that serves to increase water pressure throughout the city. Larger cities sometimes have an entire town's worth of people living and working inside one building! In skyscrapers that are taller than the average water tower, the pressure from a water tower built on the ground is insufficient. For this reason, many tall skyscrapers actually have their own water tower on the roof. They are large enough to provide water to pressurize the building's water supply and allow water to reach the top floors without threatening the pipes on the lower floors with pressure that is too high. These towers are placed at the highest point of the building because maximum elevation means maximum water pressure. While some of the water is used each day to increase the pressure of the municipal water supplied to the building, the majority of the water is held in reserve in case of a fire. Water used during high-flow periods of the day is refilled at night with a pump during periods of lower demand.

water tower, it is possible to pipe water directly to individual buildings so that it is available whenever someone turns on a faucet.

The modern water tower is conceptually similar to the ancient Roman cistern. The major difference is that cisterns were top-filled, while water towers are filled from below; but the physics behind how they disperse water remains the same. As water is raised above the surface of the earth, it gains gravitational potential energy. This energy is released in the form of kinetic energy when the water flows back down into the city's pipes at a higher velocity. In both cisterns and water towers, every foot of elevation of the water leads to increased pressure in the water. About half a pound per square inch of water pressure results from each foot the water is raised.

This added pressure is what allowed Roman cisterns to feed fountains. Pressure is required for a fountain to spray water rather than emit a slow drip. The water pressure obtained through an elevated cistern is what allowed bursts of water to come spraying out of the Roman fountains. The Roman fountain (see page 23), like many fountains still found today in Rome, gets its water pressure naturally from an ancient aqueduct that still supplies much of the city with fresh drinking water.

Modern water towers can hold about one million gallons of water, so they must be constructed with substantial support in the form of a steel frame and concrete footings. Water towers cannot be built on unstable soil and are best situated on bedrock, which can support deep foundations.

While water towers can take on any shape, most tend to be either spherical or cylindrical, and because they are visible all over town, they often become billboards for local advertisers.

LIFE WITHOUT WATER TOWERS

What would happen if a city did not have a water tower, or if the water tower were too short? Without adequate pressure, water would either slowly drip from the kitchen faucet or it might not come out at all. People living on the top floor of apartments or condominiums, for example, might not get water, while people living on the lower floors probably would.

If a water tower was too short it would be necessary to supplement the pressure advantages of the water tower with pumps at each house or building that the tower supplied with water. Though water must also be pumped up into a water tower, it is more efficient to have one large central pump than to have multiple small pumps at each building.

TOO MUCH PUMPING!

The water table is the level at which atmospheric pressure and ground water pressure are the same. It can be easily recognized as the point underground at which soil and rocks appear to be saturated.

Many cities, particularly those not located near natural reservoirs, obtain their water by pumping groundwater. However, too much pumping can lead to major problems. Consider that whenever it rains, rainwater soaks into the soil. While some of this water is absorbed and used by vegetation, the rest is forced down by gravity until it reaches the water table. This is the point where water in the ground is stable, and it coincides with the physical level at which the soil is saturated with water.

Whenever someone digs a deep well, the level of water inside the well is the same as the level of the water table. If someone dug a large number of wells on their property and started pumping out the water, their neighbors would likely have to dig even deeper for their own wells. This is because the greedy neighbor would effectively have lowered the water table in the immediate area by pumping out water at a faster rate than it could naturally be replenished.

Depression of the water table can be seen in places like Tucson, Arizona, a city that depends on the pumping of groundwater for most of its water supply. Before modern settlements, Native Americans and early pioneers used Tucson's Santa Cruz River for fishing and irrigation purposes. However, after more than 100 years of pumping, the groundwater level in the Tucson area dropped significantly, and the Santa Cruz River is now an empty channel that contains water only during brief "monsoon" storms in the summer months.

In addition to excessive pumping, people can have other negative effects on groundwater.

Groundwater supplies around 20 percent of the U.S. water supply. The protection and preservation of this resource is important. When people

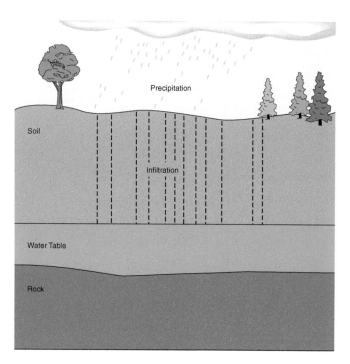

Precipitation

Soil

Infiltration

Water Table

Rock

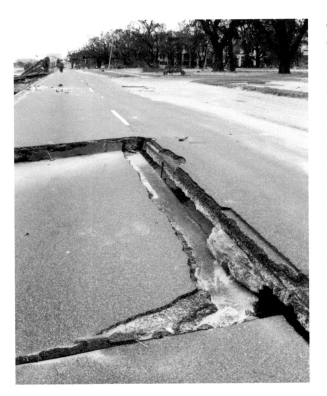

Sinkholes are created when water removes enough soil or underlying rock to create a depression, or hole, in the ground. This is an example of a sinkhole following Hurricane Katrina.

dig or otherwise disrupt the water table in coastal areas, the level of salt in the water increases because the naturally salty water found in coastal areas lies at a lower level than the fresh water that comes from rain. Also, consider that when water is removed from the soil, the soil becomes denser and more compact. This change can cause agricultural consequences that must be combated by farmers as they attempt to till and irrigate their crops properly.

Sometimes, groundwater itself causes problems. In regions where the rock under the soil is typically limestone or salt bed, this layer of rock can actually be dissolved by naturally occurring groundwater. The upper layer of soil might remain intact while the rock beneath it dissolves. Once the soil finally gives way, a sinkhole occurs. Sinkholes are fairly common in states such as Florida, Missouri, Texas, and Kentucky and are found in any area where the right type of rock exists in the natural landscape. Sinkholes can also occur when people displace too much groundwater, such as when new buildings are constructed. In these situations, local water drainage patterns are altered just enough to cause rock under the soil to dissolve or collapse. Sinkholes can be large enough to compromise roadways and damage homes and cars.

Water must be harnessed properly in order to provide for the health and longevity of people everywhere. Societies have historically found ways to divert water either to cities for personal use or to the fields for irrigation. Even water from the ground can be pumped and used for a variety of purposes. Through these different means, water is made available in the places where it is most needed.

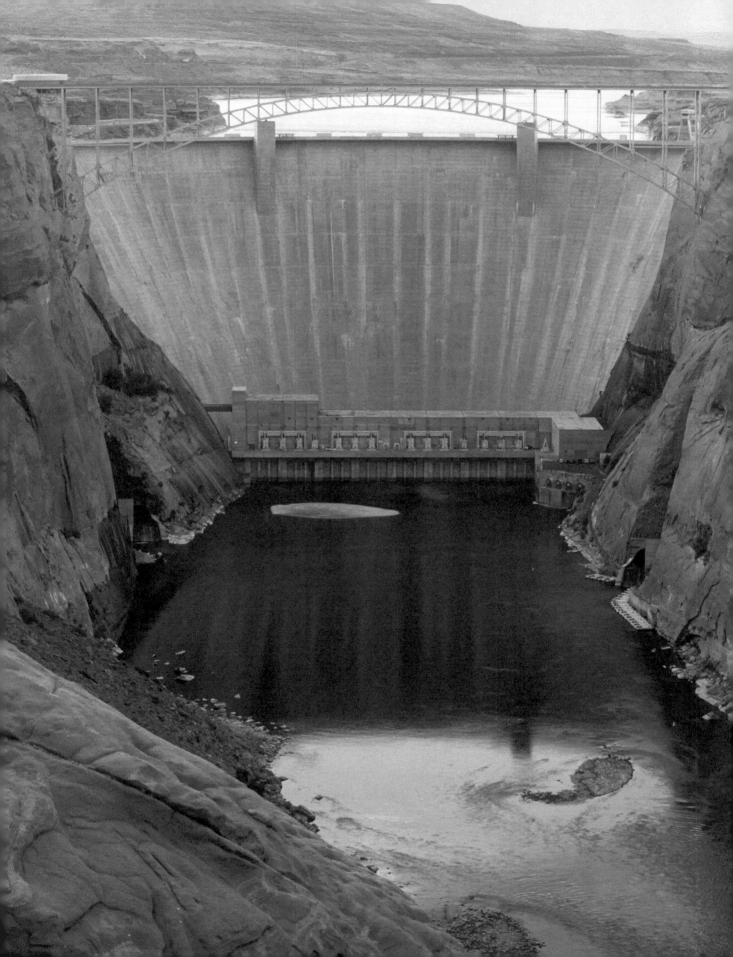

DAMS AND RESERVOIRS

Water is physically harnessed for many reasons, including flood control, steady water supply, irrigation, and even power generation. Dams alter the appearance and flow rate of water. These massive structures can have both positive and negative environmental consequences, including the long-lasting effects of their construction. However, oftentimes the environmental costs of construction are mitigated because dams have allowed for civilizations worldwide not to only exist but also to prosper.

NATURAL DAMS

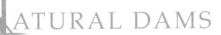

Located on the Colorado River, the Glen Canyon Dam helps store water for much of the southwest United States. Construction began in 1956 and was completed in 1966.

Humans are not the only species that builds dams. Beavers, the semi-aquatic rodents found throughout most of the United States, use their teeth to cut down trees, eat the tender bark layers, and use sticks and mud to build dams that can reach 5 or 10 feet (1.5 to 3 meters) high. Before the eighteenth century, when beavers began to be extensively hunted for their fur, their dams and the ponds they created were found all over the country.

Typically, a beaver's goal in building a dam is to create a pond that it uses for swimming and fishing. The deep pond water allows beavers to

Beavers create dams for several reasons. They serve as protection from dangerous predators, they provide an easy-to-use food source, and ecologically they help keep the local water systems intact and flowing.

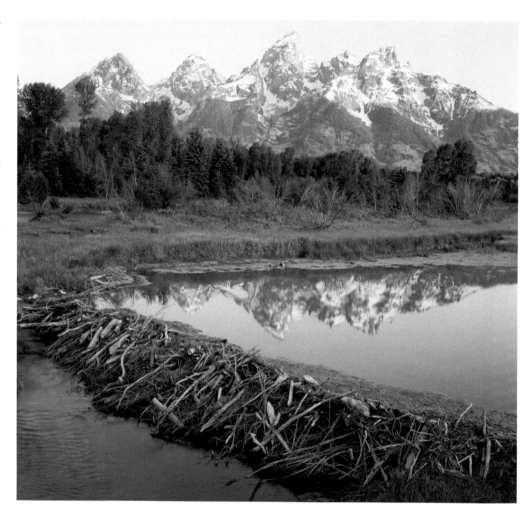

swim rather than walk when foraging for food and provides protection from predators. Beaver dams preserve water from the rainy season and release it slowly downstream throughout the year, ensuring that the stream flows all year round.

However, beaver dams have environmental consequences. They slow down the speed of rivers and streams, which reduces the kinetic energy of the water. Kinetic energy is related to the square of velocity:

$$E_k = \frac{1}{2} mv^2$$

where E_k is kinetic energy, m is mass, and v is velocity. As the velocity of the water slows down due to the obstruction, the kinetic energy is also reduced.

This slowed water speed reduces the level of erosion downstream. Water that travels faster carries more sediment along with it; slower-moving water tends to drop its sediment. When water reaches a beaver dam, the sediment is dropped into the pond while the water slowly trickles through the dam. Because of this effect, beaver ponds have a natural life cycle. They eventually become silted in and filled with sediment, and the beavers move on to a faster-moving stream to build a new dam. The pond then becomes a fertile meadow, rich with the sediment that was transported and dropped there by the stream.

FISH LADDERS

Dams can be barriers to migration. Some fish, such as salmon, swim upstream to their birthplace in order to spawn. Their travels can be obstructed by dams, so fish ladders are created to allow the fish to make their way across the artificial barrier.

Simple fish ladders can be a series of pools at different heights that allow fish to jump from one level to another. These are similar to locks on a canal that can carry boats uphill. More sophisticated fish ladders may have continuous channels leading uphill and a curved shape to save space. In areas where the vertical distance from the river to the top of the dam is very great, fish elevators can be installed. These devices use a mechanical hopper to gather fish at the bottom of the dam and transport them to the top, where they are released into a channel to swim down the other side of the dam. One such fish elevator, on the Connecticut River in Holyoke, Massachusetts, carries more than 500,000 fish per year.

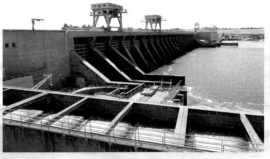

Fish ladders, or fishways, are usually built on dams or other man-made water structures. Their purpose is to encourage fish migration and breeding by allowing the fish safe passage around the obstruction.

Ice Dams

Another type of naturally occurring dam is an ice dam. These dams can form seasonally in rivers where the upstream part of the river thaws before the downstream portion. The thawed water travels downstream until it intersects the frozen blockage. It forms a pond until the river is completely thawed and the stored water is released.

Ice dams can also be formed in glacial regions. Large icebergs can break off from a glacier and block a nearby river, or the glacier itself can slowly move and end up blocking a river or inlet. Glacial ice dams can store huge amounts of water. Thousands of years ago in the Pacific Northwest, a giant glacial lake was formed by an advancing ice sheet. When the ice dam finally burst, the huge outflow scoured the landscape and produced giant waterfalls that now stand dry. It is estimated that the initial flow of water from this newly released lake was ten times the flow of all the rivers in the world!

The explosion of the Hubbard Glacier in 1986. This massive glacier is located in both Alaska and Canada, and serves as the dam that originally created Russell Lake.

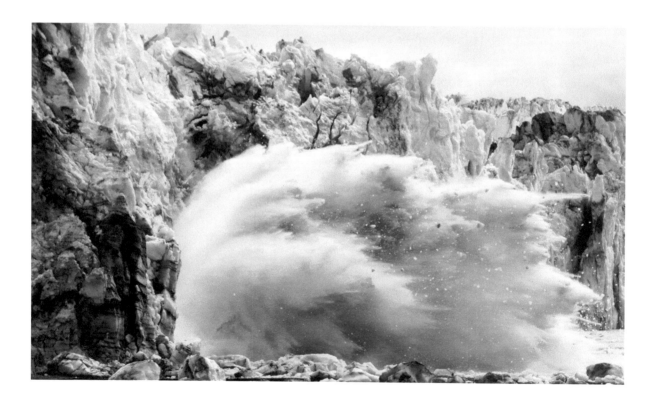

A more modern use of the term ice dam describes a ridge of ice that can block gutters on the roof of a house. As heat escapes from the house and melts snow covering the roof, the water builds up in gutters, where it is blocked by ice dams. This situation can result in leaky gutters if the ice dams are not cleared.

ANCIENT DAMS

Since ancient times, dams have been constructed to assist with irrigation and flood control. Thousands of years ago, an ancient Roman dam was built across the river Rhyndacus in Asia Minor near Aezane (now in modern Turkey). During the height of the Roman Empire, this huge dam spanned the Rhyndacus River valley and also doubled as a bridge that connected the Roman-built highways on either side of the valley. The dam, carefully constructed from huge stone blocks, featured small arches similar to those found in Roman aqueducts and bridges. These arches allowed dam engineers to modify the flow of water through the dam for flood control or irrigation. Today, parts of the ancient dam are still visible, and the positioning of a modern dam nearby illustrates how well the ancient Roman engineers selected the site.

Ancient engineers in Mexico constructed the huge Purrón Dam in the Tehuacán Valley in four stages over a period of almost 1,000 years, between 750 B.C.E. and 200 C.E. This dam was built entirely by hand, by workers who did not have the benefit of the wheel, draft animals, or metal tools. The dam had a final size of about 1,500 feet (400 meters) long, 250 feet (100 meters) wide, and 50 feet (20 meters) high. The Purrón Dam was built of stone blocks that were formed into small "rooms" filled in with rubble and dirt to provide a stable core for the dam. The dam was designed to be built and maintained over generations, and when the initial stages of the dam became insufficient due to silt deposition in the reservoir, builders simply added height to the dam. The dam was used to store seasonal water to provide irrigation for farming during the dry season.

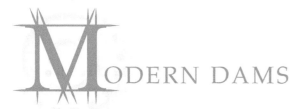

MODERN DAMS

Modern dams are based on the same principles as their natural and ancient counterparts but are much more massive in size and require sophisticated engineering to survive the forces of nature. Dams today come in a variety of shapes suited for different situations and are some of today's largest man-made structures. A dam is basically a huge wall built in the middle of a river. It must support the pressure of the river or reservoir on one side and be able to release some of that water on demand.

Four main types of dams are built today. Arch dams are thin, curved dams that are similar to arch bridges and use their shape to resist the forces of water that they must support. Buttress dams have a smooth wall on the upstream side and a series of braced supports on the downstream side. Embankment dams are huge sloped piles of dirt and rubble with a waterproof central core that does not let water seep through. Gravity dams are massive concrete dams that, like embankment dams, hold up to the forces of water pressure simply through their huge mass. Most large dams built today are gravity dams.

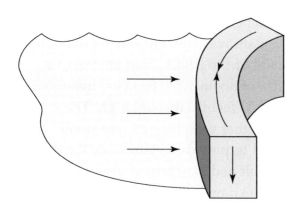

An arch dam is a curved dam. They are typically constructed of concrete and are often used for narrow rivers and gorges.

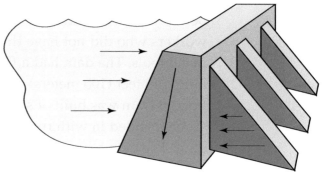

A buttress dam works like a traditional architectural buttress and is held up by visible supports. They are often built of reinforced concrete and can be straight or curved, solid or hollow.

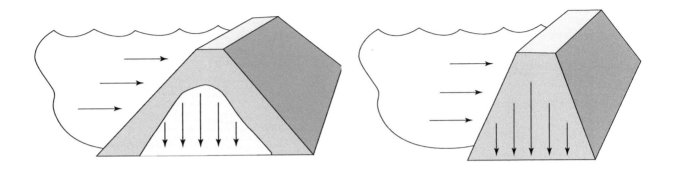

Embankment dams form an embankment against the water pressure and are typically very large, heavy dams made of soil or rock.

Gravity dams use their own weight to support themselves and can be quite large. They are useful in situations where a very large or wide water source must be dammed.

Hoover Dam

One of the largest dams in the United States is the Hoover Dam, located on the Arizona-Nevada border. Begun in 1931 and built during the Great Depression, the Hoover Dam was funded by the U.S. government as a way to provide jobs to many out-of-work Americans. Before work could commence on this mammoth dam, workers temporarily diverted the Colorado River into a series of huge tunnels blasted out from the walls of the canyon. It took workers five years to build the dam, which is 726 feet (200 meters) tall and the second highest dam in the United States. The Hoover Dam was built primarily for hydroelectric power generation, though it also served to help with flood control.

The Hoover Dam is a curved gravity dam. This design is similar to that of an arch bridge. However, while an arch bridge stands upright to counteract the force of gravity, a curved gravity dam lies down on its side with the top of the curve touching the huge wall of water it must support. Lake Mead, the artificial lake that was created upstream, pushes on the Hoover Dam. Compressive forces are created in the dam, and the walls of the canyon on either side push back and help support the structure.

The Hoover Dam is called an "arch gravity" dam because it combines the characteristics of two different types of dams. Constructed on the Colorado River in 1936, it was officially designated a National Historic Landmark in 1985.

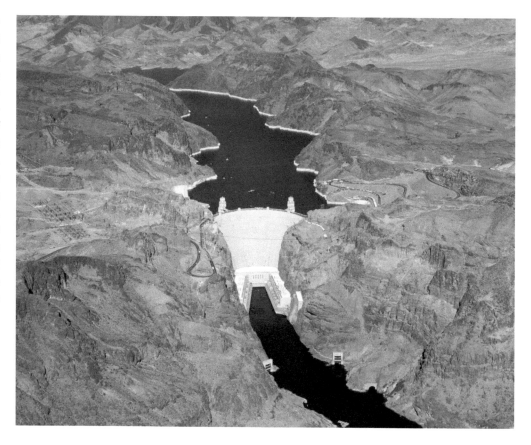

The dam is designed so that the force from the canyon walls squeezes the concrete blocks of the dam even closer together, making the dam itself more rigid and thus stronger and able to withstand the weight of Lake Mead. In fact, the Hoover Dam is so massive (660 feet, or 201 meters, wide at its base), it would be able to hold up the weight of the water even if it were not curved. Designers decided, however, that a curved design would make people living downstream feel safer because it gave the appearance of increased stability.

Aswan High Dam

Another giant marvel of engineering is Egypt's Aswan High Dam. Completed in 1970, this dam provides flood control and irrigation to the 95 percent of the Egyptian population that lives close to the Nile River. The fertile land in the Nile River valley has been farmed since the time of the pyra-

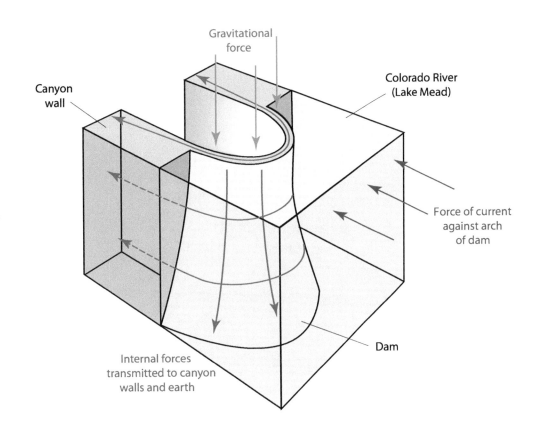

This force diagram of the Hoover Dam shows the many different kinds of forces this dam was designed to withstand. Significant forces include the weight of the water being dammed, the force of the canyon walls bordering the dam, and the internal forces of the dam itself.

Gravitational force

Colorado River (Lake Mead)

Canyon wall

Force of current against arch of dam

Dam

Internal forces transmitted to canyon walls and earth

mid-building pharaohs in ancient Egypt. The Nile River naturally floods every spring, spreading nutrient-rich soil over the farmland along the river, providing a natural fertilizer. In modern times this flooding threatened homes and businesses, and in drought years when the Nile River did not flood, farmers faced a bleak season and were unable to water their crops.

The Aswan High Dam was built to harness and control the mighty Nile River. The dam created the third largest reservoir in the world, Lake Nasser, which fills with water during the rainy season. The dam gradually releases this water for irrigation during the dry months. It also provides a large source of hydroelectric power for the region.

The dam was designed and constructed by teams of engineers from England and the former Soviet Union. It is a simple embankment dam, its basic structure consisting of a huge pile of rock and earth. This type of dam relies on its weight and size to resist the force of water pressure. In fact, construction of the dam used enough rock to build over fifteen pyramids the size of the Great Pyramid of Giza!

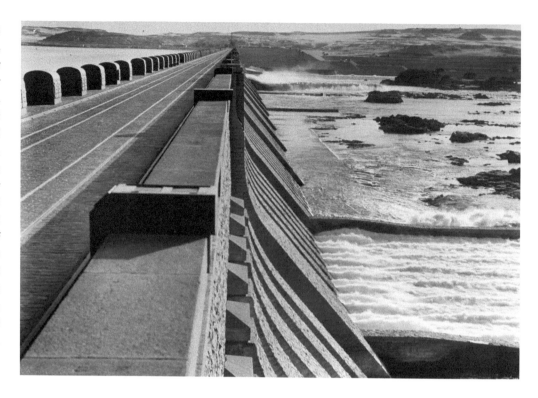

The Aswan High Dam, built for the Nile River in Egypt, was first constructed in 1902. Construction projects over the next several decades raised the height of the dam, but a second (and still higher) Aswan Dam was finished in 1970.

Unfortunately, while the dam does provide flood control and a steady supply of both water and power, the disruption of the Nile River's natural flooding cycle has had severe consequences for agriculture in the region. Normally, the sediment that was transported downstream was continually replenished with fresh fertile soil from the river's flood stages. Since the construction of the dam, that sediment has been deposited upstream of the dam when the river's velocity slows. While the reservoir is slowly filled in with silt, the farms downstream do not receive their yearly dose of fresh soil. This lack of fertilizer has resulted in a gradual decline in the agricultural productivity of one of the most historically fertile areas of the world, and farmers in the Nile valley must now use chemical fertilizers to grow their crops. While chemical fertilizers are effective, their overuse results in raised expenses and pollution.

Three Gorges Dam

A mammoth project under way in China's Hubei Province will result in the largest concrete gravity dam in the world. When finished, the dam

Constructed over the Yangtze River, the Three Gorges Dam is an astounding one mile long (1.6 km) and is more than 600 feet (182 meters) tall. These diversion locks were used during construction to divert the river around the construction site.

will be more than one mile (1.6 km) long and 600 feet (182 meters) tall and will generate more hydroelectric power than any other dam in the world. The resulting reservoir will be so large that it will be visible from space!

Such a huge project has a large impact on the environment. Already, more than one million people have had to leave their homes because the area they occupy will be covered with water once the reservoir is filled. In addition, the reservoir will cover countless ancient artifacts and fill in some beautiful canyons that are major tourist attractions. Conditions at the construction site are harsh, with workers building round-the-clock in a hazy twilight of rock dust and fumes. Environmentalists are concerned that the completion of the dam will result in the extinction of several species, including a kind of freshwater dolphin found only in the region. There is also the possibility that the dam will serve to concentrate pollutants from nearby industrial areas. However, the dam will eventually

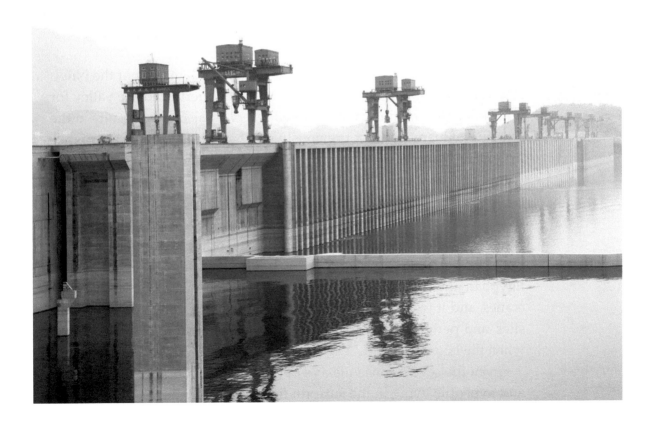

supply more than 10 percent of China's electric power and, as a rapidly growing, recently industrialized country with a finite supply of fossil fuels, China may have few other choices to meet its ever increasing demand for power.

ENVIRONMENTAL CONSEQUENCES

Dams provide many benefits to people living near them—in particular, flood control, power generation, and irrigation during dry seasons—but they also have a negative impact on the surrounding environment. These consequences can be evident immediately or over the long term, and some are difficult to predict ahead of time.

When a dam is built, it changes the shape of a river valley forever. When a narrow, unobstructed river is blocked by a dam, a large reservoir is created upstream. The purpose of this reservoir is to provide a large holding area for water, which minimizes the natural ebbs and flows of the river downstream. Water can be released from the reservoir through the dam as desired; this water can provide irrigation or be used to remove excess water if the reservoir gets too full.

Dams also have ecological consequences. The damming of the Nile River changed the natural flood cycles that had fertilized the valley for millennia. The creation of an artificial reservoir also often results in the flooding of many acres of previously inhabited land. People are displaced from their homes, and entire habitats may be destroyed.

In some cases, construction of a dam can lead to important archeological sites being covered by many feet of water. For example, in the 1960s during construction of the Aswan High Dam, engineers realized that the reservoir (Lake Nasser) would cover the site of the Abu Simbel temple built by Pharaoh Ramses II. The colossal temple was moved by the Egyptian and U.S. governments to a safe location using helicopters and cranes, and it was later reconstructed. Many less prominent archeological sites, and perhaps many undiscovered sites, were flooded with water when the lake was filled.

Given the severe consequences of dam construction to the environment and to people living in the surrounding areas, how do decision makers

The Abu Simbel temple was moved to a safe location during the construction of the Aswan High Dam.

come to grips with the negative aspect of building extremely large dams? Generally, the benefits are seen to outweigh the negatives. Most people would probably agree that careful dam construction trumps the risk of an entire city (or more) succumbing to flood or starvation.

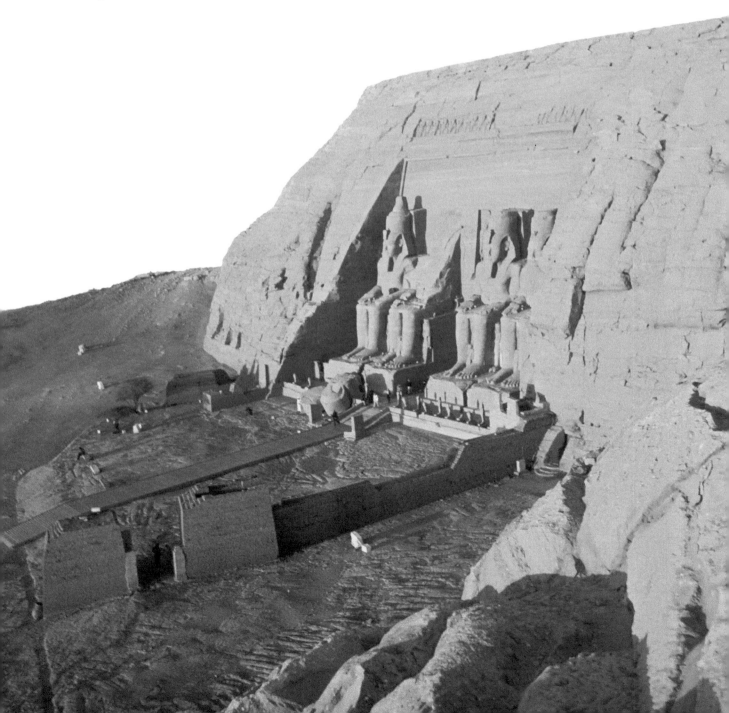

DAM DISASTER

Most failures in life have an unforeseen bright side. Flunking a test in school, for example, can feel like the end of the world; the reality is that life will go on, and you may even come out of the experience having gained new insight and determination. Dam failure, on the other hand, really can be the end of the world for anyone or anything unfortunate enough to be caught in its path. The light at the end of the tunnel is that despite the high cost of human life, engineers learn valuable information that can help prevent future disasters.

One example of a catastrophic dam failure is that of the St. Francis Dam, a curving arched gravity dam made of concrete and located near Los Angeles, California. Constructed in 1924–1926, this dam was engineered by William Mulholland and was designed to help serve the quickly growing population of Los Angeles. Mulholland had designed the 1913 Los Angeles Aqueduct, but despite the prevalence of smaller reservoirs built in the following years, the city was still in need of a large reservoir. Building a large dam to create a reservoir behind it seemed like a necessary project.

The designed capacity of the St. Francis Dam was about 30,000 acre-feet (39 million cubic meters). During the construction process, Mulholland decided to raise the capacity to about 38,000 acre-feet (47

million cubic meters), so he increased the height of the dam by 10 feet (3 meters), which made the total height 195 feet (60 meters). This additional height required the construction of a wing dike on the top edge of the west abutment. A wing dike generally serves to protect the bank of a river or creek, as well as to guide the flow of water; in this case, it was to keep water from running over the dam's edge.

In retrospect, several aspects of the dam's construction contributed to its ultimate demise. It was built on the site of an ancient landslide. Even though the land was found to be seismically safe in 1924, there was later concern that the ground was actually unstable. The dam was constructed from locally available rock, which geologists would later determine was not an appropriate material for resisting the forces of the filled reservoir. In addition, gravel from the neighboring creek bed was used for the dam without washing it first to remove the clay; omitting this washing step may have substantially altered the rock's ability to bear loads.

Cracks began appearing a year after construction was completed; more cracks were discovered when the dam was filled for the first time in 1928, and shortly thereafter the road near the dam's abutments was noticed to be sinking. Mulholland

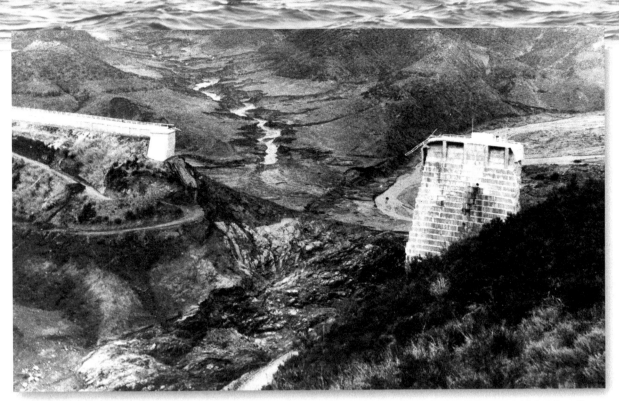

The St. Francis Dam failed completely, resulting in a tidal wave that was more than 125 feet (38 meters) high. More than 500 people are thought to have died.

continued to insist that the dam was safe, so no additional precautions were taken.

Disaster formally struck on March 12, 1928, when the dam broke apart and a massive wave flooded the San Francisquito Canyon during the dam's first full filling. The powerful water (about 12 billion gallons) felled a power station and virtually everything else in its path. The dam itself exploded into fragments that were washed away with the flood, and only the middle portion of the dam remained standing.

This flood is a prime example of potential energy. Water held behind the barrier of the dam stored potential energy, which was rapidly converted into kinetic energy as the force from the water exerted pressure on the dam (in this case, rupturing it). The water was released and rushed downstream rapidly as its potential energy (of position) was quickly exchanged for kinetic energy (of motion).

When the numbers came in, more than 500 people perished in the flood that ensued following the failure of the St. Francis Dam. That places this disaster as the second most costly, in terms of human life, in the history of California disasters. It came in second only to the San Francisco earthquake of 1906.

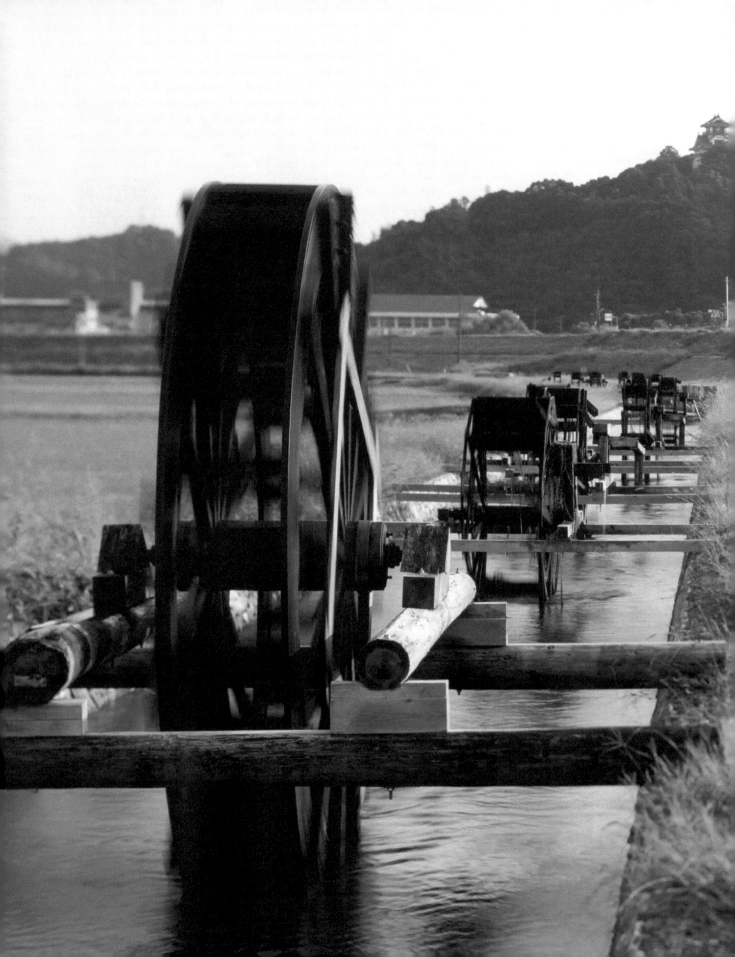

WATERWHEELS, MILLS, AND HYDROELECTRIC POWER

The use of tools to ease the daily struggles of human life is a practice that is nearly as old as civilization itself. Early humans used tools for hunting, gathering, and preparing meals. Today, farmers use plows to help till the fields, most clothing is made with the assistance of looms and other devices, and modern medicine relies extensively on technology to treat and prevent disease.

Wheels make many types of work much easier. The wheel has been around for at least 6,000 years, perhaps longer. There is evidence that in ancient Mesopotamia early humans used logs to help roll heavy objects from one place to another. Several logs at a time were used in tandem. It is thought that the wheel developed from this idea.

MECHANICS OF THE WATERWHEEL

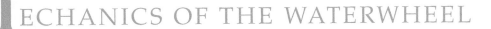

Water wheels allow irrigation using energy from the flow of the water itself.

Wheels are not only used for transportation; they can also be used to turn a shaft that does work. Beginning in about 4000 B.C.E., ancient Greek writers noted that women of the day used hand mills, or small wheels mounted to shafts, to grind grain. Around this time, one of the first machines, the waterwheel, was developed.

Traditional mills, such as this one in Virginia, used the power of flowing water to turn a large wheel, providing mechanical energy to turn a shaft that could then be used to grind grain or saw wood.

Waterwheels are fairly simple devices. A large wheel is built, and paddles are mounted to it. The wheel is placed in water that is either free-flowing or falling from some higher source. The force of the moving water turns the wheel. The main shaft, or bar that extends out perpendicular to the wheel's center, rotates along with the wheel. This rotating shaft then transmits its rotation to some other mechanical device. By this process, the waterwheel powers mills, pumps, and other labor-saving devices.

The forces involved in the turning of a waterwheel are kinetic energy and potential energy. Kinetic energy is the energy of motion, or energy derived from the speed of something as it moves. Potential energy is the energy of position—it is the energy an object has by virtue of its place with respect to external forces such as gravity. Moving or falling water

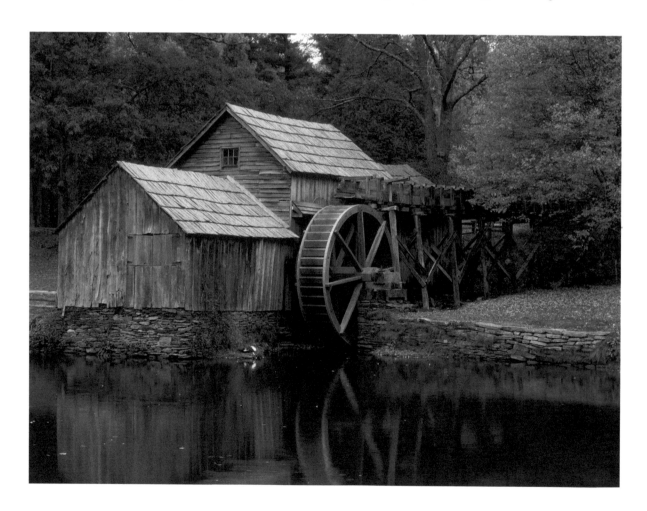

contains kinetic energy. A waterwheel contains potential energy. When the current of the water forces the wheel to turn, the potential energy of the waterwheel is converted to kinetic energy; the water essentially transfers some of its kinetic energy to the wheel and in the process slows down slightly. Waterwheels use a free and almost infinitely renewable source of energy: the motion of water!

Waterwheels are most efficiently positioned in a waterfall or a steep stream, rather than in a stream with a shallow slope. This positioning allows the wheel to take advantage of the increased kinetic energy of the water. Since water will move faster down a steep slope, the kinetic energy of the water is increased, as is the amount of energy available for transfer into the waterwheel. In situations where no natural slopes are available, an alternate solution is to pour water onto the waterwheel from an above-ground aqueduct.

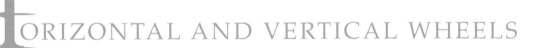

HORIZONTAL AND VERTICAL WHEELS

Waterwheels can be situated either vertically or horizontally. Early waterwheels were horizontal in orientation. A wheel was placed flat in a river or stream, and the water's current turned the wheel. The waterwheel was attached to a vertical shaft that was connected to other machinery.

Sometimes, a special chute was built to force the water from the stream into a smaller area. The chute then fed directly to the waterwheel, allowing it to turn faster than it otherwise would. This technique works well because in a stream with a constant flow rate, the volume of water flowing through one cross-section of the stream in one unit of time is constant. If the cross-section area of the stream is reduced, as with a chute, the velocity of the water has to increase to help maintain the same flow rate.

Horizontal waterwheels are much less efficient than vertical ones. There are two basic types of vertical waterwheels—overshot and undershot. Overshot wheels work by gravity: water falls from an aqueduct or waterfall above the wheel and forces the wheel to turn. Undershot wheels are generally located in a stream or river, and the forceful flow of the water turns the wheel.

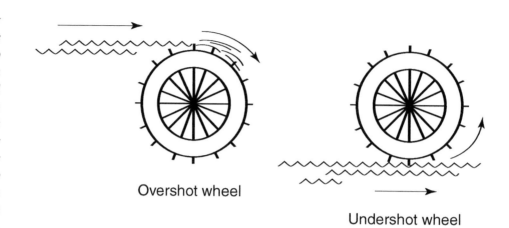

Overshot wheel

Undershot wheel

Vertical water wheels can be designed to turn with water supplied from above, in the overshot wheel, or through water moving below the wheel, in the undershot wheel.

Vertical waterwheels also take up less floor space than those that are oriented horizontally. However, if the only mechanical work that the watermill needs to produce is something that involves a vertical shaft, then a horizontal wheel may be easier or more convenient to use.

WATERWHEELS BEFORE ELECTRICITY

One of the most important uses for a waterwheel is in irrigation. A waterwheel connected to an informal system of canals forces water out into the fields. This system even allows water to travel to fields that may be higher in elevation than the water source. Waterwheels are also useful for pumping drinking water to various parts of a village.

In the eighteenth and nineteenth centuries, as industry grew, the waterwheel was used to run gristmills, sawmills, and other machines. A gristmill is a building to which grains are taken from the field and ground into flour. The mill typically had a large waterwheel on the outside, which was connected to a flatter wheel inside the building. Grains were ground into a fine powder and distributed for sale. In sawmills, lumber was cut down to size for use in construction or other applications. In early sawmills, the waterwheel would provide a continuous source of power for the saw blade. When metals became more readily available as building materials, waterwheels also powered mills for cutting and lathing metal sheets.

The water-wheel's motion turns a shaft inside the mill. Depending on the application, the motion of the shaft can be changed in direction using gears such as bevel gears, or split to turn multiple shafts located else-where in the mill using belts.

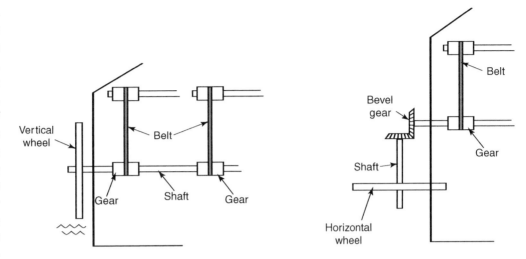

Textile mills also used waterwheels, though they were slightly more complicated and involved more mechanical parts. The earliest textile mills appeared around the end of the eighteenth century on the East Coast of the United States. They typically had a waterwheel with a shaft that was connected to several large gears. Each of these gears was then connected to the rest of the machine by a belt. Long belts allowed the energy

IN GEAR

Gears are mechanical devices that aid the transfer of force in machinery. The distance between the center of the gear and the place where the gear contacts another object is known as the gear ratio. Gears usually have teeth or ridged edges that connect with other gears, and all generally lie flat in the same plane. Bevel gears have straight or spiral teeth, and the teeth themselves have angled edges. The gears are connected to cylindrical shafts that are placed at 90-degree angles to each other. Because the shafts for two interlocking bevel gears are perpendicular to each other, bevel gears change the direction of rotation by 90 degrees.

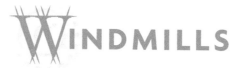 Windmills

Windmills are traditionally used as a way to generate energy from the wind, but they can also be used to help pump groundwater. In rural areas that are not typically connected to the city's power grid, water-pumping windmills are the most efficient way to produce water for irrigation.

A windmill is any machine that converts wind into energy. Windmills typically have a number of blades attached to a rotor. When the windmill's blades encounter wind, they turn. This rotation provides mechanical energy for whatever other machinery the rotor is connected to, and the purpose of this machinery is to perform some type of work. Historically, this work has involved tasks like moving a big stone to grind grain.

The energy generated by the turning of the blades can also be used to pump water. To do this, the rotor is connected to an underground pump. This pump removes groundwater from the soil and usually stores it in a holding tank for later use. In some cases, the windmill may be located directly over a well, which is simply a verti-

cal hole that has been dug down to the level of an underground aquifer. Groundwater is present at a particular depth beneath the surface known as the water table, and below this depth the ground is saturated with water, so it is easy to pump from it.

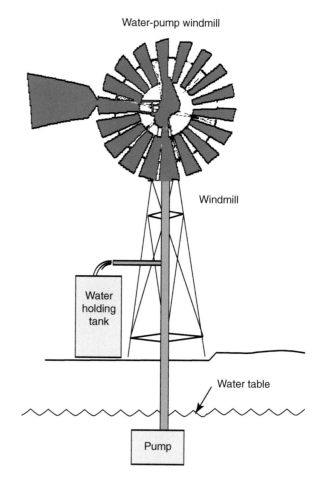

The wind turns the blades of a typical windmill, which allows a pump to pull water from a well hole drilled below the windmill down to the water table. The water is drawn up when sufficient wind blows and is stored in a holding tank for future use.

The efficiency of a windmill is determined by a number of factors: the size of the blades and rotor, how windy an area the windmill is placed in, and the strength of the water pump. Generally, the energy from a windmill can be seen as a function of the diameter of the rotor and the speed of the wind:

$$E = 0.0109 \, D^2 V^3 x$$

where E is the energy generated, D is the rotor diameter, V is the wind speed, and x is the strength of the pump.

The amount of energy that is generated (and the amount of water that can be pumped) varies tremendously depending on these factors. Since the pump and rotor are consistent from day to day, the wind speed has the greatest influence on the total energy generated. Since the wind does not blow all day every day (or at the same times of day), water pumped from windmills is best used for crop irrigation or water for livestock. Water for humans must be 100 percent reliable and consistent!

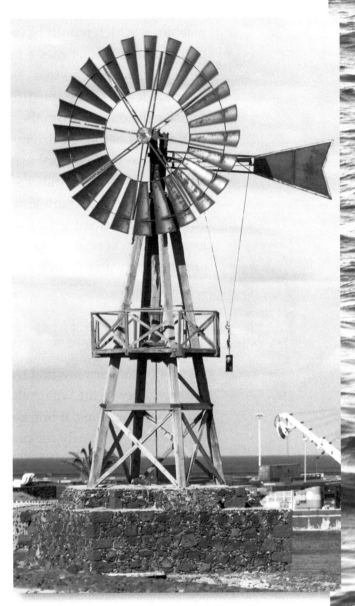

This windmill, in Spain's Canary Islands, is used to both generate electricity and pump water.

from the wheel to be directly transferred to the weaving and spinning machines, which would have been located some distance away, inside the mill building. Sometimes a horizontal waterwheel was used to generate power for the mill. In this case, bevel gears (gears that fit together at a right angle to change the direction of rotation) would have been used to transfer the energy from the wheel into the machinery.

In the era before electricity was available, mills allowed people to operate big, heavy machinery using water as the power source. The disadvantage of this was that mills could be built only in locations where there was a river with enough kinetic energy to drive the machinery. With the advent of electricity, manufacturing centers like mills could suddenly be located anywhere: urban and industrial areas no longer relied specifically on a nearby water source for their power.

HYDROELECTRIC POWER

The major modern method that harnesses water power, and is based on the principles of the waterwheel, is hydroelectric power. Many of the world's major dams, while also built for flood control or drinking water, are intended primarily for power generation through hydroelectric power.

The basic principle of hydroelectric power is that electricity can be generated from the motion of water. The primary piece of equipment used in generating hydroelectric power is a hydraulic turbine—a machine that functions much like a propeller. The turbine is a direct descendant of the waterwheel.

A hydroelectric power station begins with a dam. Water that flows from the dam, usually located some distance above the actual turbine, contains a great deal of gravitational potential energy due to its height. Once it falls into the turbine area, the water turns the blades of the propellers, which are part of an assembly

In a turbine generator, electricity is generated when water moves over the blades of a fan-like turbine. This motion turns a shaft, which then turns a rotor. Magnets in the rotor move around a stationary conductor such as copper, inducing an electric current that can then be harnessed as electricity.

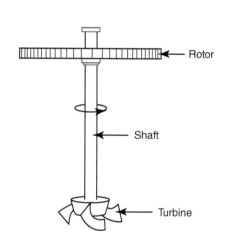

Rotor

Shaft

Turbine

Giant turbines, such as these in the Grand Coulee Dam power plant, are used to transform the motion of water over a dam into electricity.

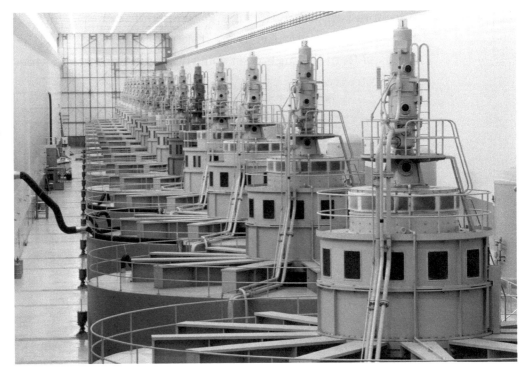

called a turbine. The turbine is connected to the shaft, which is then connected to the rotor; the entire upper assembly is called a generator.

When used in a power plant, the flow of water turns the rotor of the generator, thus generating power. Enormous magnets in the rotor turn inside stationary copper coils. An effect called electromagnetic induction takes place when a conductor, like the copper coils, moves through a magnetic field like the one generated by the magnets in the rotor. In this case, the copper is stationary and the magnetic field moves with the rotor. This setup creates an induced electric current in the copper coils. The kinetic energy of the moving conductor is converted into the electrical energy of the flowing current. The current is converted with a transformer into the type of power that is needed for consumer-based electricity. Power lines then carry the electricity generated at the power plant out into the community, where the power is dispersed as needed.

One common variation on the hydroelectric power plant is a pumped storage plant. This kind of plant contains two separate reservoirs, one located at a high elevation and one located much lower. Water is pumped from the low reservoir to the high reservoir during off-peak hours, where it is stored and ready for use. When people demand more electricity (when everyone returns home from work, for example), the water is released from the high reservoir and spins the turbines, thereby generating electricity.

Benefits of Hydroelectric Power

Hydroelectric power generation has existed in the United States for about 120 years. The first hydroelectric power plant was located in Wisconsin near the Fox River, and opened for business in 1882. Since hydroelectric

RENEWABLE ENERGY

Most of the energy produced in the United States still comes from fossil fuels or nuclear power. Hydroelectric power is a clean and renewable alternative. It is certainly much cleaner than coal, which was the only electric power source before hydroelectric. It is also considerably less expensive than fossil fuels; the price of water does not increase like the cost of a barrel of oil. While hydroelectric power in the United States is limited to about 8 percent of total power production, worldwide that figure is more like 23 percent.

There is, however, a downside to the use of hydroelectric power. Constructing large dams has a negative environmental impact, as they certainly change the ecology of the region and can have devastating effects on the local community if they break. Ecosystems in the water around the dam will change, potentially causing disruptions to spawning fish or other wildlife. Also, the physical disruption of the turbine in the water can alter the composition of the riverbank and riverbed.

Occasionally, if a dam is large enough, people living near the building site have to give up their homes and move elsewhere.

power requires running water, plants tend to be located near rivers, waterfalls, or dams. Waterfalls are convenient, but do not offer a way to store water for later use. Rivers are also convenient, but without special interventions it usually is not possible to control how fast the water flows into the turbine. Dams require a significant initial construction cost, but they offer a stable, consistent supply of water for a hydroelectric power plant.

Currently, most hydroelectric power plants for the United States are located in the northwestern states of California, Oregon, and Washington. China generates much of its electricity by hydroelectric power, as do Canada and Brazil. Countries with lots of mountains and waterfalls, such as Switzerland, also tend to make extensive use of this free, efficient natural resource.

A major benefit of hydroelectric power is that electricity can be generated nearly constantly. Especially when using dams, water is always present. There is no reliance on the procurement or delivery of fuels. Because dam water is stored, it can be used at any time, and hydroelectric power plants can generate more power during peak hours (and less during nonpeak hours). There are no waste products to be disposed of, and water-based power plants do not pollute the air. Also, when compared to other alternative energy sources such as wind or solar power, hydroelectric power is consistent and reliable. In fact, the Hoover Dam generates more than 4 billion kilowatt-hours of power every year, enough for 1.3 million people.

Water has the potential not only to sustain life, but also to make life easier and more convenient for people. There are various ways to harness the power of water and turn it into functional energy, and people have been researching and developing these methods for hundreds of years. Waterwheels and hydroelectric plants use a renewable source of energy to make thousands of daily tasks possible.

Sawmills

Hydro-powered sawmills, particularly those from the seventeenth and eighteenth centuries, were an elegant example of how the motion of water could be harnessed for a specific, mechanical process. A sawmill has a straightforward purpose: push a log into one side, and receive lumber (construction-ready wood that has been cut to a specific size) out the other end. What happens in between is where it gets interesting!

The beginning of the process for turning logs into lumber remains more or less the same today. Logs are felled (cut down) and sized to a rough length. They are then hauled, either by truck, train, or river, to the sawmill. Somewhere along the way the logs are also scaled, which means they are graded based on length and weight to determine the volume of wood contained in each log. Once they get to the mill, the logs are sorted, de-barked, and roughly cut so that they will fit into the mill blades. They are then cut to size, trimmed to ensure that they have square ends, dried, planed, and delivered to distributors so that the lumber can be sold.

The "original sawmill," which consisted of two people working together to cut a log using a whipsaw, required extensive manpower and time. The addition of a water-

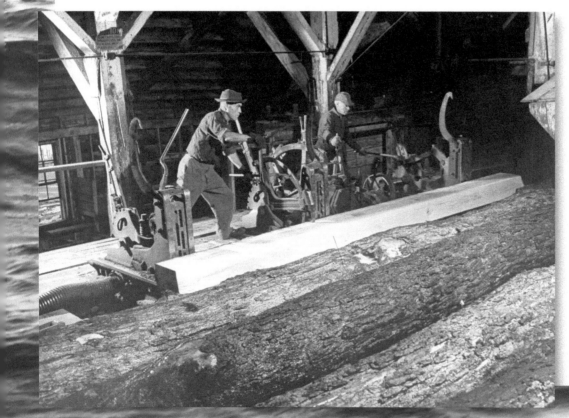

Old-fashioned sawmills relied on the expertise and abilities of its workers.

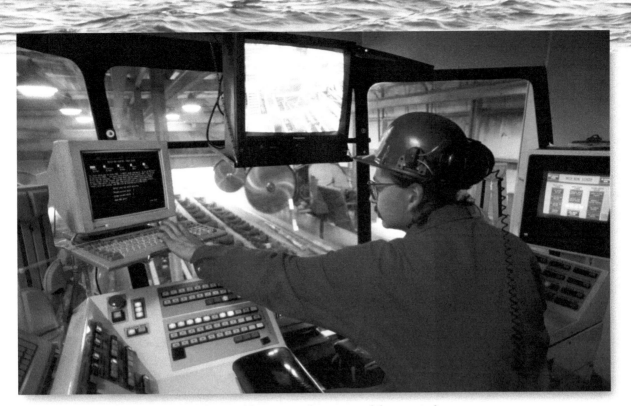

Modern sawmills use computer technology and lasers to perform many of the same tasks.

wheel to power the whipsaw led to immediate savings in time and energy. Sawmills initially used water to power only the saw blade itself; workers stood behind the logs and manually pushed them into the saw. Ancient writings reveal that water-powered mills may have been in use as early as the fourth century B.C.E., and they were a common sight on the landscape in the years to come. Ancient hydro-powered sawmills were used throughout Europe, Africa, and Asia.

A major improvement to the sawmill design came with the invention of a motorized sled that carried the logs through the blade at a consistent pace. Many more improvements followed, including the use of multiple blades, which made short work of converting logs into dimensionally sized lumber. Nineteenth-century innovations in steam technology, which used water in a

different capacity from a waterwheel, allowed sawmills to be larger and more powerful (in addition, of course, to not having to be built on a river!).

While some modern sawmills are powered by gasoline, most are run using electricity. In fact, most of the work that was previously done by skilled workers is now automated by computer systems. In years past, sawmills generated a substantial amount of "wood waste." Chippings, shavings, and sawdust abounded as by-products of the lumber creation process. Mills today gather these castoffs and use them to form "wood products" such as compressed wood, wood pellets, paper, OSB (oriented strand board), fiberboard, and particleboard.

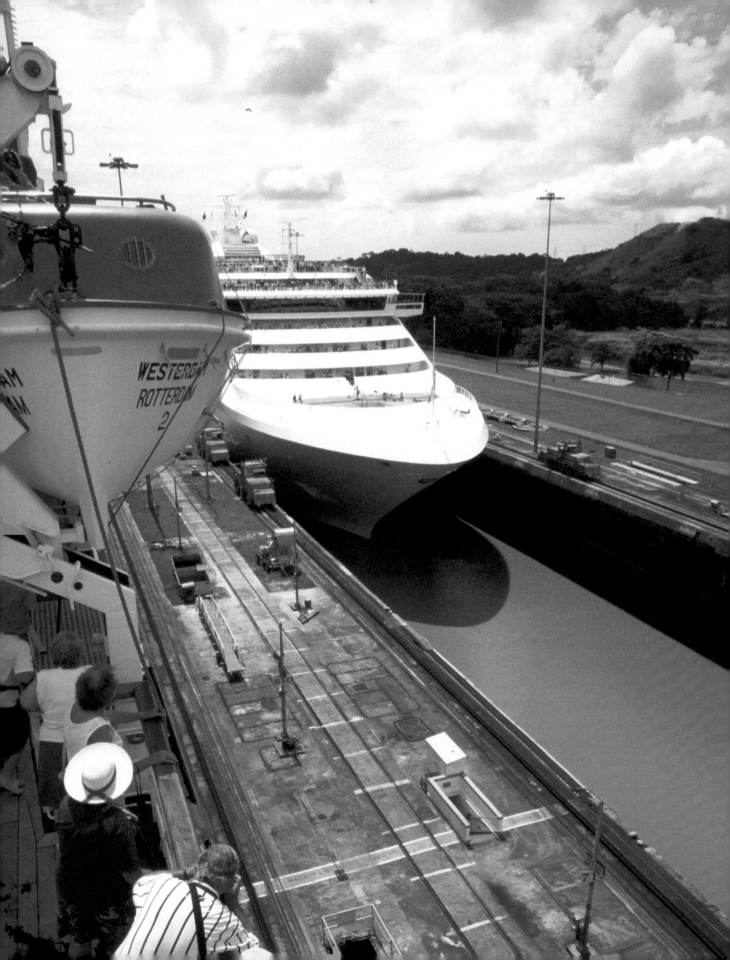

TRANSPORTATION CANALS AND LOCKS

The Panama Canal is just large enough to allow huge cruise ships to pass from the Atlantic to the Pacific Ocean. In fact, the size limit on the design of many new cruise ships is that they have to be narrow enough to pass through the Panama Canal.

One of the most important uses for waterways is to help people to travel from place to place. Water was one of the world's primary sources of transportation for generations and remains an important method for moving passengers and freight.

The starting and ending points of any journey across an ocean or down a river are predetermined by natural boundaries. Passengers traveling down a river on a rafting trip, for instance, can choose from a range of destinations that the river flows past. Ocean travelers must have departure and destination points along the coasts. However, throughout history people have often wanted to travel to other destinations not located near rivers or other convenient bodies of water. When food or other equipment had to travel from one place to another and there was no available river going in that direction, man-made waterways were sometimes created.

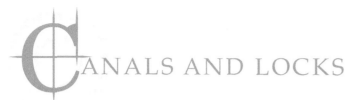CANALS AND LOCKS

A canal is a man-made, or artificial, water passage. Canals can be created from scratch or they can be extensions of existing rivers. They are used for transportation and for irrigation and often connect two larger bodies of water. These natural sources usually supply the water that fills the canal. Canals can also be built as artificial branches from rivers that extend out to surrounding areas.

Boats can easily navigate through canals that are flat and straight, but sometimes canals must travel through areas where elevations change. Boats have trouble with large changes in elevation, so locks were designed to allow boats to successfully travel through canals that experienced changes in slope or height due to the surrounding terrain.

A canal lock (which can also be used in rivers) is a physical construction that helps lift or lower a boat between changes in water level of a canal. Locks generally operate as a platform or enclosed chamber with gates on each end. The gates help control the water level inside the locked portion of the canal, and this change in water level is what lifts or lowers the boat.

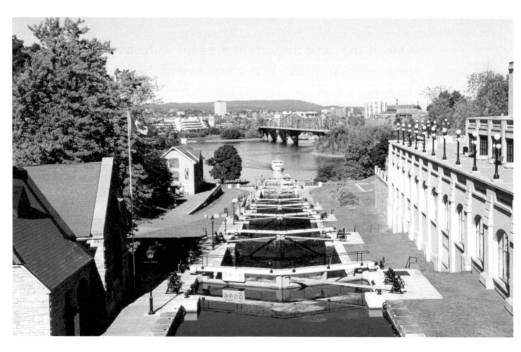

Locks, such as these historical step locks on the Rideau Canal near Ottawa, Canada, allow a boat to change levels to enter a body of water lower or higher than its initial position.

DAMS AND WEIRS

Some canals incorporate dams and weirs to control the flow of water. If the water level in a canal or river is too low to allow large boats to travel, a small dam can be built across the river. Water builds up behind the dam until it flows over the top. Such an overtopped dam is called a weir. Weirs artificially reduce the flow rate of the canal, causing more water to build up in a certain stretch of the canal and therefore deepening the water level. This process can allow larger boats to travel in that section of the canal. Such a process can be repeated downstream, resulting in a canal with a number of deep pockets of water, each bounded by a weir at the downstream end.

While weirs allowed boats to travel small sections of a canal, they created the problem of how to allow boats to pass from one section of the canal to another. An ancient technique was called the flash lock. This is a device such as a door or gate in the middle of the weir. Opening the lock door releases water so that it flows downstream. As water rushes out through the lock, ships are carried "downstream" along with the water. The flash lock, an early precursor to the modern navigational lock, was in use as early as 50 B.C.E. in China. The release of water from the upstream portion also served to free any boats that might have become trapped in shallower portions of the downstream section of the canal. However, the method was dangerous due to the rapid release of water, and many boats capsized and sank.

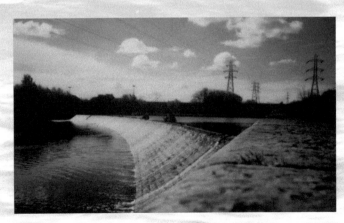

A weir, such as this one, is a low overflow dam that serves to raise the water level behind it.

Since water flows under the force of gravity, it attempts to create an equipotential surface that is at a constant elevation. When a canal is built that must incorporate changes in elevation, water would naturally flow down an open channel and eventually empty the canal. Locks are artificial barriers that keep this from happening. When the gates are closed on the lower section and opened on the upper section, water flows into the lock and fills it to the height of the upper section, thus forming a flat surface. Entering from the lower section, a boat or other object floating on the surface of the water is raised to this new level. Once the water levels reach equilibrium (balance), the boat continues its course at the new, higher level. A similar method is used to allow a boat to travel from a higher elevation to a lower one within a canal.

EARLY CANALS

Canals have been used for irrigation since the earliest days of farming, in places such as the Nile River valley in Egypt. More sophisticated canals, which allowed for navigation, became common in the Middle Ages in many parts of Europe, particularly in countries near to or bordering on the ocean. There are many canals in the Netherlands. Many Dutch settlers earned their living by fishing or farming, and canals were useful in both occupations. One of the earliest canals was created in Delft, Holland, around 1100 C.E.

Canal du Midi

One of the oldest canals in southern France is the Canal du Midi, built in 1681. The canal is about 150 miles (240 kilometers) long. It varies in width, with an average distance across of 60 feet (18 meters). The original purpose for the Canal du Midi was to provide a connection between the major seas in the region—the Atlantic Ocean and the Mediterranean Sea. During the late seventeenth century the open seas were overrun with pirates, so a safer method for moving freight and goods was needed. In addition, the journey around Spain was expensive due to taxes imposed by the Spanish, and the 1,800-mile (2,900-kilometer) journey was long and

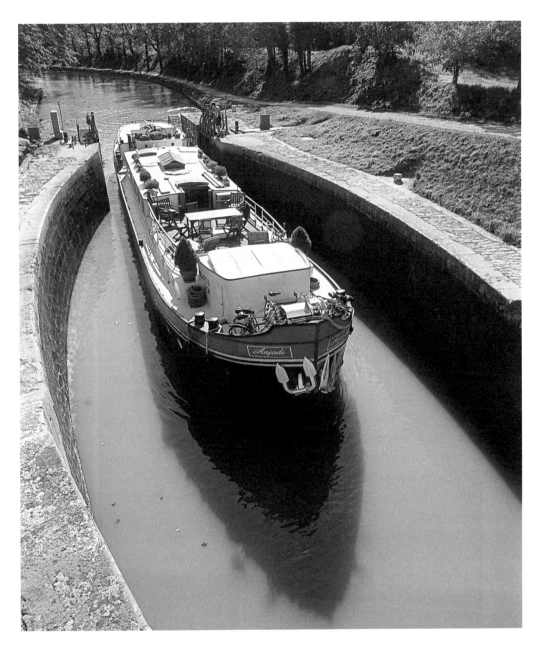

A ferryboat traverses the Canal du Midi in France.

arduous. The Canal du Midi provided safe, inexpensive passage for merchant ships.

A tax collector named Pierre-Paul Riquet spearheaded the canal project. He obtained approval from King Louis XIV, and the project began but ran out of funding before the canal was completed, and the engineer ended up having to spend his own money. The Canal du Midi was an

GRAND CANAL OF CHINA

Some of the best and most fascinating constructions in the world were built long before our time; the Grand Canal of China is one. It is the longest canal from antiquity and carries with it a rich tradition of Asian building and history. In fact, it is both the oldest and longest canal in the world and is much larger than either the Panama or Suez canals.

The origins of the Grand Canal can be traced back to the fifth and sixth centuries B.C.E., when powerful warlords established that a canal could benefit trading between states, in addition to keeping warriors stocked with supplies. The first portions of the canal, those connecting the Huai and Yangtze rivers, were actually created from lakes, rivers, and other existing water sources. Later dynasties added on to the canal, with the same basic goals: fuel the military, increase trade, and transfer needed goods (like grain) to the capital.

The Grand Canal has a massive total expanse of about 1,115 miles (1,794 kilometers), spanning the distance between Hangzhou and Beijing. However, the shorter navigable portion runs between Jining and Hangzhou and is divided into seven separately named canal sections. The canal currently includes over sixty bridges and twenty-four locks.

China's Grand Canal has historically been used to transport food, supplies, construction materials, and trading goods from distant locations to the bustling city of Beijing. It also provided an efficient means of moving people from place to place, which allowed for the intermingling of cultures and the spreading of political doctrine. In that sense, the Grand Canal was a simultaneous source of both unification and diversification for this large, spread-out country.

The total vertical elevation change across the length of the canal is about 126 feet (38.5 meters). Most rivers in China tend to flow from west to east, so the general north-south trend of the Grand Canal allows connections to be made between river valleys such as the Yangtze River valley and the Yellow River valley.

The canal was built primarily by unskilled peasant laborers. During the political unity of the Sui Dynasty, principally during the years 605–610 C.E., Emperor Yangdi built up a labor force of over 6 million peasants to link the canal from the agricultural regions in the south to the capital, Beijing, in the north. Unfortunately, over half of the 6 million men working on the canal are said to have perished, leading to the downfall of the Sui Dynasty in 618 C.E.

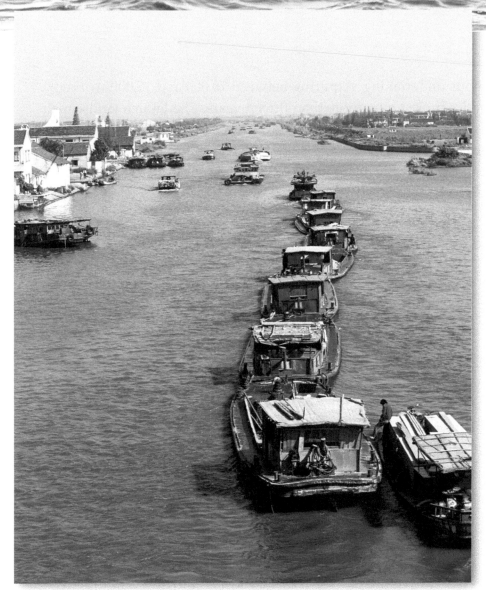

The Grand Canal of China is the longest canal of the ancient world, spanning 1,115 miles (1,794 kilometers). It plays a central role in sustaining many aspects of Chinese life and culture.

However, the cultural changes brought about by the canal did serve as an overall uniting force, ushering in the stable Tang Dynasty (618–907 C.E.) during which China emerged as a powerful country.

Today, the Grand Canal still exists in many locations. It is currently being restored to its former glory in some regions as a way of diverting water, and many parts are navigable and used for shipping, fishing, and recreation. Like the Great Wall of China, the Grand Canal remains as an impressive accomplishment of a past civilization that still stands, and is used, today.

enormous undertaking, requiring between 10,000 and 15,000 workers. The entire project took more than fifteen years. The French landscape is far from flat, so the canal required sixty-three separate locks. A number of bridges and a tunnel were also constructed. The tunnel was bored through the Malpas Hill and is notable because it was one of the first sea tunnels to be constructed in Europe.

ERIE CANAL

In the nineteenth century, as the United States grew, it became clear that travel by foot or pack animal was not the most efficient means for moving resources around the country. New York was one of the largest commercial areas, but many precious resources (wood and minerals, for example) were located miles away. A trip from New York to the Midwest on horseback took weeks under the best weather conditions, and much longer in winter.

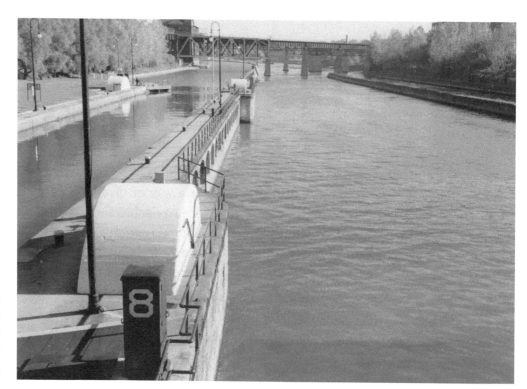

The last lock on New York's Erie Canal before it enters Lake Ontario.

THE RAILROAD VERSUS CANALS

The Erie Canal made it easier and faster to transport goods between the Great Lakes and New York. For years the canal was the only practical way to ship things such a great distance. Later on, railroads competed with the canal for business.

Steam-powered train engines did not appear in the United States until 1826. The locomotive developed rapidly around this time, and commercial railroad tracks appeared steadily over the next twenty to thirty years. Once railroads were in place, they became very popular for moving freight because of the fast speeds at which locomotives could travel. Shipping using the railroad was, however, much more expensive than the Erie Canal, so the canal continued to see heavy traffic. The canal system was enlarged and dredged a number of times over the years, and in 1918 was reopened as the New York State Barge Canal. However, railroads and highways gained in usage during the first half of the twentieth century, and commercial canal traffic dropped substantially after the 1959 opening of the St. Lawrence Seaway. Today, the New York State Canal System is used primarily by private recreational boats.

New York's Governor DeWitt Clinton proposed a solution to the problem of transporting resources across America: a canal that would connect Lake Erie directly to the Hudson River. Though the idea had been considered as early as 1700, research into its feasibility began in earnest around 1800. Clinton championed the building of the canal, pointing to the success of similar canals in Europe. The idea was approved and funded by the New York State Legislature in 1817.

The Erie Canal was planned to be 363 miles (584 kilometers) long with an average width of 40 feet (12 meters). It was built with more than eighty locks. Though detractors were quick to dub the canal "Clinton's Folly" and "Clinton's Big Ditch," it opened for business in 1825 and had an enormous impact on the country's economy. Now that trade between the Great Lakes and New York City was possible, more and more settlers headed west. The fertile land in the west allowed newly arrived farmers to grow large amounts of crops and sell them back east for a tidy profit.

The Erie Canal is an impressive feat of engineering, which was not an official profession in the early nineteenth century. There were no "certi-fied" engineers to supervise the design and construction. Literally thou-sands of maps were drawn of the canal and its surrounding landscape, and new roads had to be constructed in order to move people and tools to the canal site. Most of the digging was done by hand, as power tools and excavators were not yet available to aid in the process. In areas where the canal was to be dug through solid rock, blasting powder was used to create tunnels that workers refined manually.

Suez Canal

One of the most important canals in Eurasia is the Suez Canal, which runs through Egypt and connects the Mediterranean Sea to the Red Sea. The canal allows for freight passage between Europe and Asia; previous-ly, the only way to move goods between these destinations was to ship them around Africa.

The Suez Canal was built on the site of an earlier canal, dating to the period of the Egyptian pharaohs (c. second century B.C.E.). This ancient canal was repaired many times over the centuries, but the creation of a new canal was not formally undertaken until the mid-1800s. The Suez Canal project was a multinational event: it was financed by both Egypt and France, used Egyptian laborers, and was designed by an engineering team from Austria. Construction began in 1859.

The project was politically charged from the very beginning. Because the British were dominant in the region and did not want a French canal to threaten their business interests, the British persuaded the Egyptian workers to rebel, thereby ceasing work efforts on the canal. Construction was eventually restarted, and the canal was open for business by 1869. Despite its rocky start, the canal became immensely popular for moving goods between countries.

Another political crisis occurred in 1956 when the Egyptian government nationalized the Suez Canal Company. The president of Egypt had been denied loans from the Americans, British, and French, and decided that taking ownership of the canal might help raise revenue for Egypt. The canal was closed for several months during foreign-led invasions in the ensuing Suez crisis, but eventually reopened for business in 1957.

It was not necessary to construct locks for the Suez Canal because it runs through terrain that for the most part is flat. Its total length is 101 miles (163 kilometers), and it varies in width. The canal has one shipping lane with several so-called passing bays, which are similar to the turnouts

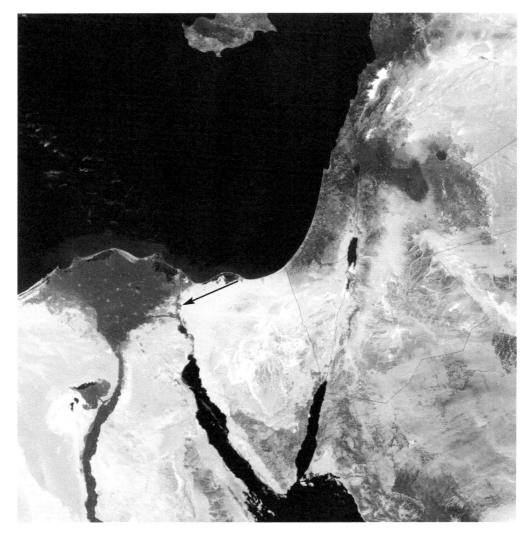

The Suez Canal, in Egypt, connects the Mediterranean Sea (top) to the Gulf of Suez (middle), which leads to the Red Sea (bottom). The Nile River is to the left of the Suez Canal.

seen on winding mountain roads. Passing bays are inlets specifically designed for one ship to pull aside while another ship passes it.

One interesting fact is that because the water of the canal is not very deep, extremely large ships cannot pass through every section. To get around this problem, the canal company leases ships that can get through. Larger vessels can offload some of their cargo to one of these ships, which allows the larger vessel to pass through the shallow water. The cargo is then retrieved at a point further down the canal that is less shallow.

Ships float in water because they are buoyant. This means that the ship is pushed upward by a force equal to the weight of the water that it displaces. The level at which a boat floats in water depends on the boat's weight, its density, and the shape of its hull. The amount of the boat that is below the surface of the water is called the draft. Large or heavy boats may have a deeper draft, which can make them unable to navigate shallow channels, such as parts of the Suez Canal. Removing some of the ship's cargo onto a second local ship reduces the mass of the large ship, and helps it float at a higher level. The draft of the ship is reduced, and it can then navigate shallower channels.

PANAMA CANAL

Most canals are built to solve a specific problem, and the Panama Canal is no exception. The idea of cutting a canal through Panama to connect the Atlantic and Pacific oceans first came about in the early sixteenth century. The Spanish government discussed building a water passage as a means to expedite exploration, but the idea remained dormant until the early 1800s. Once news of the 1848 California gold rush made it to Europe, Spain in particular expressed further interest in building such a canal.

A French company (led by Ferdinand Marie de Lesseps, the same person responsible for the building of the Suez Canal) made further evaluations, calculating that at least 17,500 miles (28,160 kilometers) would be saved on round-trip travel between the coasts of the United States if a waterway were constructed through Central America. Previously, transport from the East Coast to the West Coast of the

United States had to go all the way around the southern tip of South America, which took months.

The U.S. Congress conducted a formal inquiry. Once the route through Panama was determined, the United States signed a contract with Panama that ensured a permanent lease on the canal zone. Construction began in 1881 and was completed in 1914.

The Panama Canal spans about 51 miles (82 kilometers) and is interspersed with artificial lakes, dams, and three major locks. The building of the Panama Canal was one of the most difficult engineering projects of all time. By its very nature, building a canal is physically challenging work. While some dredging equipment was available, the Panamanian landscape was filled with large rocks that were quite difficult to move. By 1904 steam-powered equipment was brought to the site by the Americans, greatly increasing the workers' productivity. In addition, locks were eventually used as a way to avoid having to dig the canal so deep in some areas.

More than 27,000 workers died during the construction process. There was insufficient health care for the workers, and many succumbed to tropical diseases that are prevalent in the region.

The Panama Canal does not rely on external power sources. The dams are used to generate electricity, which is then used to open and close the canal gates and run the locks. The Panama Canal is an interesting example of a self-contained system: hydrothermal power is collected from the motion of water over dams, and this power is then used to operate other aspects of the canal system.

Canals are an efficient means of transporting people, animals, and goods from one place to another. Their construction is arduous, and often takes dozens of years, thousands of workers, and millions of dollars. But the benefits reaped from a canal last for centuries. Even today, when airplanes and trains are common conveniences, canals are still used to transport the largest and heaviest items.

THE PANAMA CANAL EXPANSION PROJECT

There is an old expression that "water will find a way." Find a way it will, but sometimes humans have to give that water a little push in the right direction. Such is the case with the Panama Canal, which for years has been in need of expansion in order to accommodate more traffic, as well as to keep growing as a major part of the world's maritime transportation network.

The Panama Canal Expansion Project, also known as the "Third Set of Locks Project," has been in the works for more than seventy years. Studies and projections confirmed that if Panama Canal cargo traffic and volume continue to grow at their anticipated rate, the canal would need to be able to accommodate larger and heavier vessels.

The project itself consists of adding a third lane and the necessary lock chambers. These locks will be three-chambered and gravity-fed, meaning no additional pumps will be used. Planned dimensions would be 1,400 feet (427 meters) in length, 60 feet (18.3 meters) deep, and 180 feet (55 meters) wide. One set of locks will be added on the Pacific side of the canal, and another on the Atlantic side. The anticipated construction timeline could allow the new locks be used by as early as 2014.

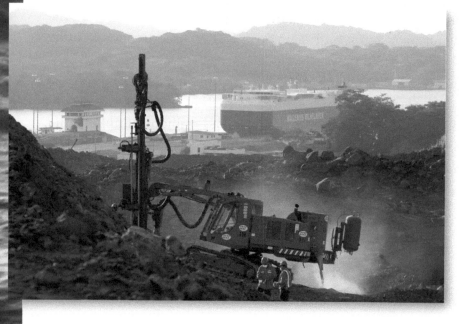

The new locks proposed as part of the Panama Canal Expansion Project will be as environmentally friendly as possible, utilizing rolling gates and boat-driven vessel positioning.

FOSSILIZED CANALS

Irrigation canals were used in prehistoric southern Mexico to allow farmers to grow crops year round. Canals and irrigation structures built up to 3,000 years ago are still visible in some areas near Mexico City. Canals in the Tehuacán Valley spanned a distance of more than 745 miles (1,200 kilometers) and provided irrigation water for 127 square miles (330 square kilometers) of land. Even though these canals were initially just small rock-lined trenches built in the soil, many of them still exist today due to the high mineral content of the water in the region.

The canals of Tehuacán diverted water from springs in the region that had a very high concentration of dissolved minerals. In particular, these waters had large quantities of a type of calcium carbonate called calcite. In rapidly flowing rivers or streams, the calcite stayed in solution in the water, but when the water was diverted into shallow, slower-flowing irrigation canals, the calcite came out of solution and crystallized into a thin layer on the bottom and sides of the canal.

The crystallization was largely due to the evaporation of water from the canals, which increased the concentration of calcite in the remaining water. Changes in temperature and pressure as the water flowed out of the springs into the canals probably contributed to crystallization. The process of crystallization is similar to what happens in caves where stalactites are built up over time by water with a high mineral content. As layers of the calcite were deposited in the canals, they built up and hardened into a rock-like layer called calcareous travertine. In a typical canal, up to a centimeter of travertine could be deposited each year.

It may seem that travertine would fill in the canals completely. But the coating was also deposited on the outside of the walls of the canal, which caused the walls to harden and rise above ground level. Over centuries of use, the canals built up into ridges that could be 100 feet (30 meters) wide and 13 feet (4 meters) high. These ridges had a working canal at the top, high above the ground level. The properties of the travertine mean that even after the canals were abandoned in the 1500s, they remained visible in many regions. The fossilized canals are known as *tecoatles,* which means stone snakes in the Aztec language.

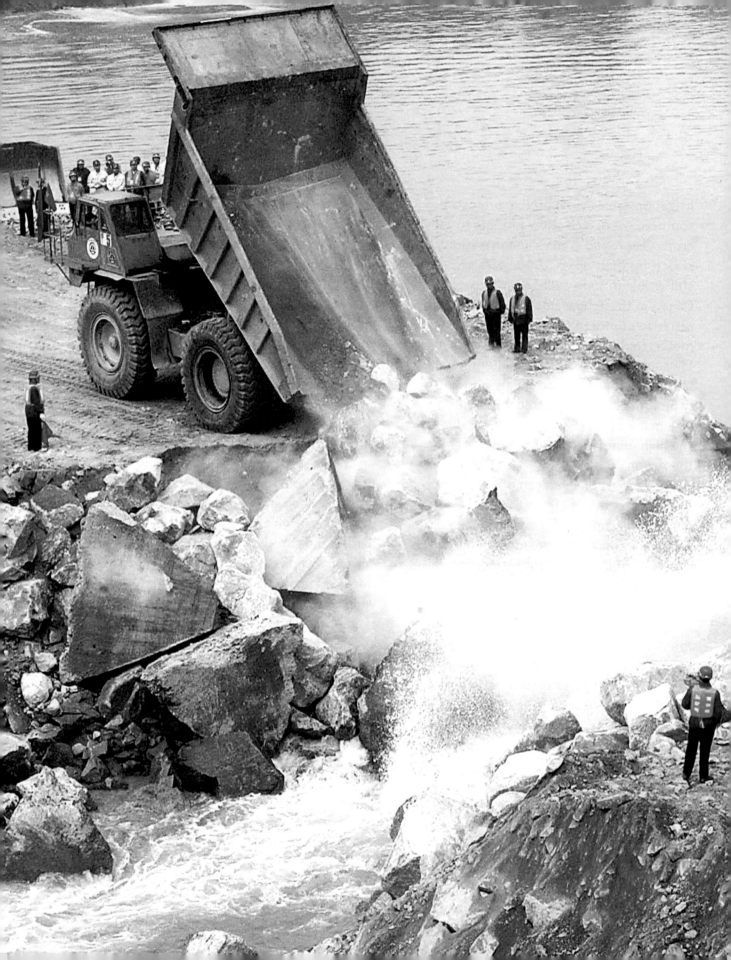

PROBLEMS IN RIVER ENGINEERING

River engineering is the science of intentionally diverting or otherwise influencing the course of a river, usually to benefit humans in some way. River engineering has been practiced ever since human populations began building civilizations near rivers.

Unfortunately, things do not always go the way engineers plan. Mistakes are made, sometimes on a grand scale. The consequences of such mistakes vary, depending on the scale of the project and the size of the error.

DA VINCI'S DIVERSION OF THE ARNO RIVER

The construction of China's Three Gorges Dam required the damming of the mighty Yangtze River.

One of the earliest examples of river engineering gone awry occurred during the Renaissance. Leonardo da Vinci (1452–1519) is best known as one of the most important artists of the period. But da Vinci was also an anatomist, sculptor, architect, and inventor. His notebooks reveal sketches for some of the world's firsts: he designed a bicycle, an armored tank, a fortified castle, and a hang glider, among many other inventions.

Da Vinci also had a hand in river engineering. His interest turned toward the Arno River, which is a major river that flows through the

Tuscany region of Italy. The Arno flows into the Ligurian Sea, the northern arm of the Mediterranean, and is not easily navigable. Renaissance Italy was not a particularly peaceful place, and various Italian city-states were constantly defending themselves against attackers or attacking others to gain land and power.

Da Vinci lived in Florence in the early sixteenth century and served as both a political and military advisor to the ruling families. He believed that the Arno River could be diverted to run behind the city of Pisa and flow directly from Florence to the sea. He designed a canal system that could carry boats and goods for trade, provide military access to far more areas, and also serve as a national irrigation system. Da Vinci's partner in this endeavor was none other than Niccolo Machiavelli (1469–1527), one of the best-known philosophers and political writers of the period.

Da Vinci's plan, had it succeeded, would probably have made the independent city-state of Florence a full seaport and major super power. He gathered a team of several hundred workers and, under the guidance of his chief hydraulics engineer, work on the main canal system began. Unfortunately, when Leonardo had to leave to continue another project, the canals took a disastrous turn. Ditches were dug in the wrong places, there was a massive manpower shortage, and a flood ultimately prevented the completion of the canal. Interestingly, a highway that has been constructed from Florence to the sea follows the path Leonardo had so carefully researched and drawn.

Leonardo da Vinci's sketch of the Arno River, including his plans to divert it.

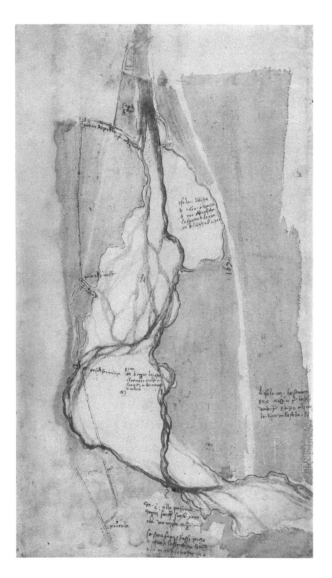

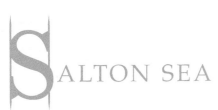ALTON SEA

One of the more disastrous stories of river engineering is that of the Salton Sea. In 1901, irrigation canals were dug from the Colorado River in an attempt to aid with irrigation into the Imperial Valley in southern California. The main goal of the Imperial Canal was to divert enough river water to help create usable farmland in this part of the country, which is typically hot and very dry.

The California Development Company started construction, but it quickly became apparent that the canal was not of sufficient strength, size, or quality to meet the original goal. It quickly became filled with far more silt than had been anticipated, and much of it was soon blocked. Engineers attempted to rectify the problem by releasing more water from the Colorado River into the Imperial Valley, but this proved disastrous when heavy flooding in 1905 ripped through the canal and began flooding the Salton Basin.

Since water will take the easiest path to the lowest accessible elevation, the Colorado River adopted the new canal as its new route. Once the

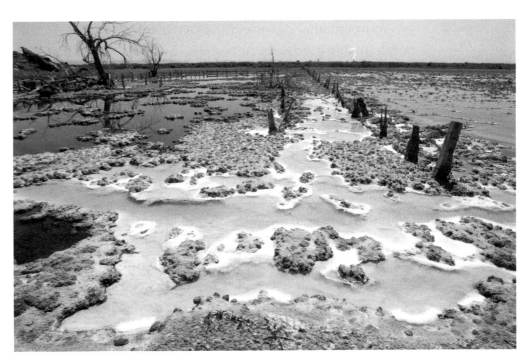

White salt crystals are visible in brines from the Salton Sea, which have flooded a near-by farm. The Salton Sea has gotten saltier and less habitable since its accidental formation.

river had found its new channel, the entire flow of the Colorado River began flooding into the valley. The sheer volume of water that was flowing into the valley made it extremely difficult to stop it—imagine the kinetic energy of an entire river!

It was not until 1907, when a boulder levee was built along the break in the river, that the river's new path was finally stopped. By this point, a huge lake had formed, measuring about 40 miles by 13 miles (64 by 20 kilometers) dubbed the Salton Sea. The valley contained an amount of water equal to the entire output of the Colorado River over two years. It flooded the farms and homes in the area, causing residents to flee.

Salty Sea

In an attempt to salvage something from the situation, the area was turned into a fishing and recreational area. However, an artificial lake with no inlets or outlets will quickly begin to evaporate, removing the fresh water and leaving behind salt and pollutants. The salt level of the Salton Sea began to rise almost immediately, but it was sufficient for many breeds of fish to thrive for the first few decades.

After a century of evaporation, however, the Salton Sea is something of an environmental debacle. It has a considerably higher salt level than the ocean, making it nearly impossible for most fish to survive. The average salinity of the ocean is 35,000 parts per million (ppm). This means that the ocean is 35,000/1,000,000, or 3.5 percent, salt. By comparison, the salinity of fresh water is less than 1,000 ppm. The salinity of the Salton Sea is close to 44,000 ppm, or 4.4 percent salt, and the number is still increasing.

Why is the Salton Sea so salty? Water evaporates quickly in hot, dry climates, leaving any salt in the water behind. This means that the original amount of salt is now contained in a smaller amount of water. There is no fresh water running into the Salton Sea except for the occasional rainfall, so it gets saltier and saltier as time passes.

The Salton Sea is also highly polluted due to runoff from nearby agricultural areas that use pesticides. Unlike natural lakes and ponds, the Salton Sea does not have a source of clean water to help dilute the contaminants. The sea is home to an unusually high concentration of sick wildlife, particularly birds, and the fish that still live there may not be

PRECIPITATION

If water is constantly evaporating from the earth's oceans, what prevents them from drying up completely? The answer lies in precipitation. Rain, snow, sleet, and other types of precipitation form continually in clouds, which are created from condensed water vapor in rising air. Some estimates place the time between water evaporating and then condensing as rain to be around eleven days. The rain falls directly on the oceans, as well as onto land, where it drains into lakes and rivers. Much of the surface water eventually makes its way to the oceans, where it evaporates again. This phenomenon, known as the "water cycle," helps explain the general balance of life on Earth.

safe to consume. As the Salton Sea has no runoff, selenium resulting from sewage and other contaminants reside in the bottom of the lake, where they become part of the food chain. The Salton Sea area is an unpleasant place to visit, and it bears little resemblance to the recreational area that was first envisioned.

FAILURE OF TETON DAM

Another example of a spectacular failure was the Teton Dam. This federal project was originally developed to cross a large canyon over the Teton River near Idaho Falls in southeastern Idaho. It was intended to provide power, serve as a flood barrier, help irrigate the surrounding areas, and create a recreation area. The design called for a dam measuring about 3,200 feet (975 meters) long and rising more than 300 feet (91 meters) out of the water.

Several locations were studied for the site of the dam. Test holes were drilled into the rock and showed that some seepage would possibly occur if

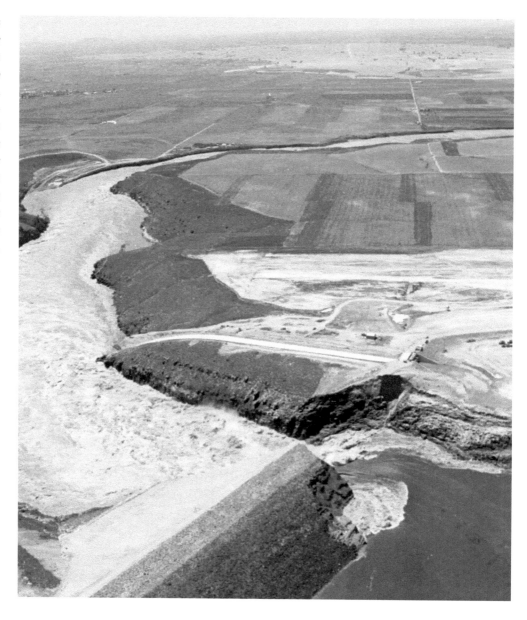

Water rushes through the ruptured Teton Dam in Idaho on June 5, 1976. The ruptured dam is clearly visible in the lower middle, with the rushing waters to the left of the break.

the dam were built along the canyon. Geologists studied many sites in the area and came to the same conclusion about each of them. However, construction was eventually approved by the U.S. Army Corps of Engineers, and the dam was built between 1972 and 1976. It was designed as an "earth fill embankment" dam, which meant it was built largely of earth.

Approximately 10 million cubic yards (7.6 million cubic meters) of earth were dug up from the reservoir bed and used in the construction of the dam. Workers also used gravel, cobblestones, clay, and sand. The earthworks were firmly pressed down, and layers of rock were added on top of the earth base. The foundation for the embankment had several major components: trenches 70 feet (21 meters) deep were dug along the abutments, a cohesive layer of foundation grout was installed, and rock was excavated underneath the actual abutments.

Unfortunately, the Teton Dam failed before it ever had a chance to prove its usefulness. Generally, in order to construct a dam, cofferdams (underwater enclosures) are built to divert the water both above and below the future location of the dam. In addition, diversion tunnels are used to guide the river water away from the dam site for the duration of construction. This temporarily exposes the dry riverbed at the dam site so the dam can be constructed. In the case of the Teton Dam, once construction was complete, engineers began slowly allowing water to fill in behind it. As the dam began to fill over several days, several small spots of water seepage were observed, but these were not considered unusual for a dam constructed largely of earth and silt. On June 5, 1976, as engineers were preparing to fill the dam to capacity, a major leak developed at the north abutment. The flow probably started as a leak, but eventually turned into a disaster, with water flowing out at 50 cubic feet (1.4 cubic meters) per second. Water began leaking from more locations, and engineers were unable to fill the gaps.

A whirlpool had begun forming in the reservoir, and it increased in size over the course of the morning. The hole in the dam got bigger and bigger, and eventually the embankment fell into it. By the end of the day, almost half of the embankment was destroyed, and the reservoir was completely drained. Fourteen lives were lost. The $100 million spent on the project was wasted, and nearly three times that amount would be spent by the government in lawsuits relating to the dam collapse. Most of these lawsuits came from cities located miles downstream from the dam that were flooded.

Causes of the Dam Collapse

The U.S. Bureau of Reclamation was assigned to investigate the cause of the failure. The main possibilities were poor construction, inappropriate or low-quality earth materials, or a flaw in the design. No single cause was ever pinpointed by the bureau. One of the more likely theories points to cracks in the dam as the major contributing factor.

How could a small crack be responsible for the complete failure of a dam? A look at the theory of crack propagation offers an explanation. First, the energy needed to initiate a crack is much larger than that needed to continue the formation of the crack. Once that initial activation energy is reached, it is relatively easy for a crack to continue to expand. A crack in a material will continue to grow larger if the energy required for the crack to expand (E_c) is equal to or greater than the material's resistance to the crack (R):

$$E_c \geq R$$

As long as the change in energy causing the crack exceeds the material's capability to resist it, the crack will continue to grow until the material breaks. In the case of the Teton Dam, the pressure of the water exerted force on the material of the dam. Eventually the activation energy was

THE TETON DAM

The Teton Dam embankment was constructed in five different zones. These zones were created to specify different layers of materials and, since the basalt and rhyolite rocks found by geologists at the site were not typically thought to be structurally sound for a dam of this magnitude, these zones were a necessary and integral part of the construction.

Zone 1: central core, silt
Zone 2: core and seepage protection, gravel overlay
Zone 3: downstream stability, fill
Zone 4: upstream cofferdam, fill
Zone 5: outer rock fill

reached, and the water found a small zone of weakness in the dam that it could exploit to begin a crack. Once the small crack formed, more and more water tried to force its way in, providing sufficient energy to continue expanding the crack until the entire dam failed catastrophically.

BANQIAO RESERVOIR DAM

The 1975 failure of the Banqiao Reservoir Dam, located in the Henan Province of China, was one of several that resulted from a major typhoon. The flooding caused by this dam breakage was extreme, resulting in thousands of deaths.

Flooding in the Huai River basin had been a fairly regular occurrence for years. In the 1950s, the Banqiao Reservoir Dam was built in response to this flooding. It was also intended to help generate power for the region. The dam was about 380 feet (116 meters) high and, despite some early cracks that were repaired with help from the USSR, it was considered one of the strongest dams of the day. It was designed to withstand what was referred to as a 1,000-year storm, and for a time the dam fulfilled this goal.

What the builders of the dam did not count on was the onslaught of a 2,000-year storm, which came in the form of Super Typhoon Nina in 1975. The storm began as a tropical depression, or a cyclone with relatively low wind speeds, but quickly turned into a typhoon. Cyclones are low-pressure areas with strong winds that originate in the tropics, progressing from tropical depressions to tropical storms to full-fledged cyclones. They are further subdivided into hurricanes and typhoons, depending on which ocean they originate in.

At its peak, Typhoon Nina reached wind speeds of up to 150 miles per hour (241 kilometers per hour). When the warmer typhoon air combined with a cold front from the north, the rain and wind exerted hefty forces upon the dam, and the sluice gates could no longer contain the flood of water. During this period, nearly a foot of water per day was storming down. Ironically, the government had granted permission to open the dam in an attempt to relieve some of the pressure, but the message did not make it to the dam operators in time.

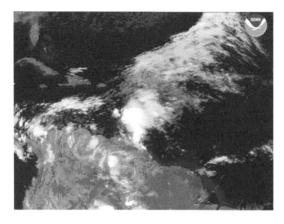

Top: A tropical depression in the Caribbean. Note the lack of structure.

Middle: Tropical Storm Ernesto heads toward Florida. This storm type is stronger and more organized than a tropical depression.

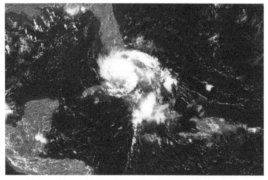

Bottom: Hurricane Katrina heads toward New Orleans. This strong hurricane had winds of 175 mph (282 km/h) and was organized into a spiral shape with a central eye.

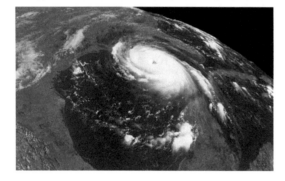

Eventually, both the Banqiao and its neighboring Shimantan Dam reached capacity. As the floodwaters rose above the crest of the dam, the water burst through the dam and caused it to collapse. The reservoir water combined with the excess from the previously collapsed Shimantan Dam upstream, and 780 million cubic yards (600 million cubic meters) of water passed through Banqiao Dam. A massive wave was generated, measuring between 10 and 20 feet (3 and 6 meters) high and nearly 6 miles (9.5 kilometers) wide. Much of the surrounding Chinese countryside was flooded as more than sixty smaller dams also burst in the storm. The impact on human life was enormous. In order to prevent the same fate from befalling many of the region's other dams, some were forcibly destroyed by the military to guide the floodwaters into more viable areas.

Combined Flooding

Why would one dam affect the flooding of other dams? Consider that when floodwaters are pouring downstream at a very fast pace, they quickly combine with the reservoir waters that a dam is retaining. If the dam fails unexpectedly, that reservoir water is immediately added to the floodwater, and the combined water volume forms a larger problem that continues to make its way downstream.

TYPHOON FREQUENCY

What is a thousand-year storm? Meteorologists who predict the weather classify storms in terms of relative frequency per year. Big storms are less common than smaller storms. A particular type of small storm might take place a few times a year while a more intense storm might only take place once every few years. A storm with a relative frequency of 50 percent will take place, on average, every two years. The highest classification of storms is usually a Class 5 extreme storm. This type of storm has a relative frequency of 0.1 percent, meaning that on average one will occur approximately every thousand years. Of course, such a statistical definition is no guarantee that there will not be two thousand-year storms in a row, but such an occurrence would be extremely unlikely!

Dams are usually built as static structures, made to support the pressure of a wall of nonmoving water contained peacefully behind them. The situation changes dramatically, from a physics point of view, when a dam breaks upstream. In addition to the weight of the static water that the dam was built to support, the dam must now contend with the force exerted on it by a large wall of water rushing downstream from the broken dam site. The kinetic energy of this water is as follows:

$$E_k = \tfrac{1}{2}\, mv^2$$

where E_k is the kinetic energy, m is the mass of the extra water, and v is the velocity of the water. When a dam breaks, the potential energy of the water behind the dam is represented as:

$$E_p = mgh$$

where E_p is the potential energy, m is the mass of the water, g is the acceleration due to gravity at the surface of the earth, and h is the height of the water.

In this case, the height h corresponds to the height that the water was held above the regular level of the river by the dam that broke. The potential energy of this water, before the dam breaks, is equal to its kinetic energy after the dam breaks, converting the excess height into velocity as the water races downstream.

$$E_k = E_p: \frac{1}{2}\, mv^2 = mgh$$

$$\text{Solve: } \frac{1}{2}v^2 = gh$$

$$v = \sqrt{2gh}$$

Since g is a constant, we can easily figure out the initial velocity of the water from its initial height above the river level in the dam.

TYPES OF STORMS

Cyclone: A storm system that originates in the tropics. Cloud circulation travels counterclockwise in the Northern Hemisphere and clockwise in the Southern Hemisphere. A cyclone is defined as a rotating system of storms and wind, fueled by heat released from condensing water vapor.

Tropical Depression: A system of clouds and thunderstorms with winds less than 38 mph (62 km/h).

Tropical Storm: A system of sustained thunderstorms with winds between 39 and 73 mph (62–117 km/h).

Hurricane: A tropical cyclone that originates in the Atlantic Ocean, with winds greater than 74 mph (118 km/h). This type of storm has a defined circulation structure with an eye in the middle.

Typhoon: A tropical cyclone that originates in the Pacific Ocean, otherwise similar to a hurricane.

Once the water reaches the second dam downstream, it will impact the dam with this kinetic energy. Velocity might increase as the water proceeds downstream, especially if the gradient is fairly steep between the two dams, or it might decrease due to friction along the riverbed. In any case, its velocity will still be significant when it impacts the second dam.

Since the second dam must suddenly support not only the weight of the water that it usually has in place but also the new wave of water from upstream, it is very likely to crack or rupture under this onslaught. Once there is sufficient energy to form a small crack, it is much easier to continue the crack and requires less energy to sustain it. It is likely that the Banqiao Dam collapsed due to just this set of circumstances.

Failures in river engineering can be nearly as spectacular as achievements. Whether through poor planning, incorrect calculations, or the fury of Mother Nature, dams and canals always have the possibility for failure. Because the consequences of such failures tend to be extreme, modern structural designers generally err on the side of caution, over-engineering where possible. Flood-protection devices are not only beneficial, they can save lives.

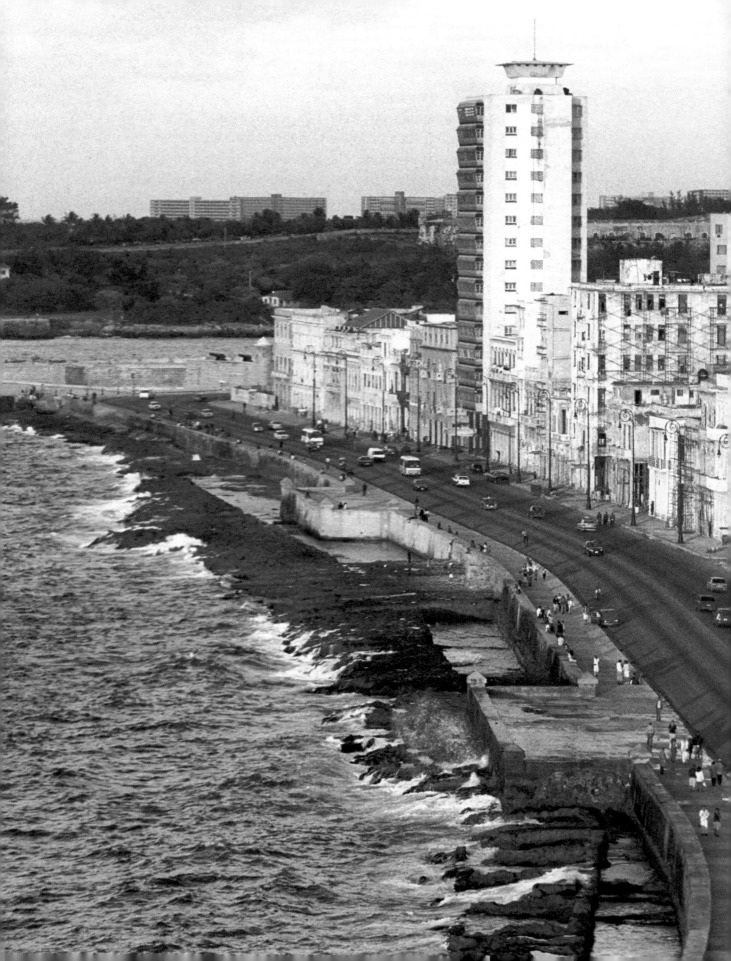

FLOOD PROTECTION

Living near water provides many advantages, ranging from irrigation to transportation, but with these benefits comes an increased flood risk. Dams and canals can provide some protection, but engineers have also created structures specifically designed to prevent flooding. Geography is a major factor in deciding the most appropriate method of flood control, and local building traditions are also an important consideration.

Dikes, levees, seawalls, and flood barriers can range in complexity from a simple earthen wall to a complex system of mechanical gates. Unlike dams or canals, seawalls and levees have more flexibility in the nature of their construction. These alternate flood-protection devices are usually permanently installed and function all the time, though some may be activated only when water reaches a certain level. This enhanced flexibility allows engineers to control flooding in the most effective way possible.

DIKES

Cuba's El Malecon seawall protects coastal buildings from the ocean.

The oldest type of flood protection system is the dike. The classic execution of this type of flood wall is seen in the Netherlands, where a vast system of ancient and modern earthen walls keeps back the sea and prevents the land (which is below sea level in many places) from flooding. The landscape of the Netherlands is quite flat, and the average elevation of much of the land is only about 3 feet (1 meter) above sea level.

Human activity is responsible for the low elevation of Dutch land. Over the centuries, swampland at relatively high elevation was drained by settlers and converted into farmland. This drainage dried out the underlying peat, causing it to compress and lower the level of the land. Residents then had to lower the groundwater level even further by increasing the drainage to maintain their farmland, causing the peat to compress even more. Centuries of this practice have resulted in a country that is under severe threat from the sea.

Beginning in about the twelfth century, residents started to band together, constructing large walls to protect their farmland from flooding. As the ground level continued to drop, an organized system of dikes emerged. An important part of this system involved windmills, which pumped groundwater out of vulnerable areas. Lakes were drained to create more usable land.

In 1953, a huge flood killed 1,835 people and resulted in a government plan to try to control the sea, thereby protecting Holland from future floods. The construction of a massive series of dikes, called the Delta

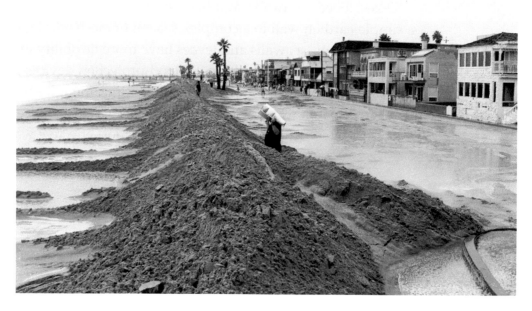

A sand dike protecting a beach in Orange County, California. This simple mound of sand and dirt keeps the ocean from inundating the homes near the beach.

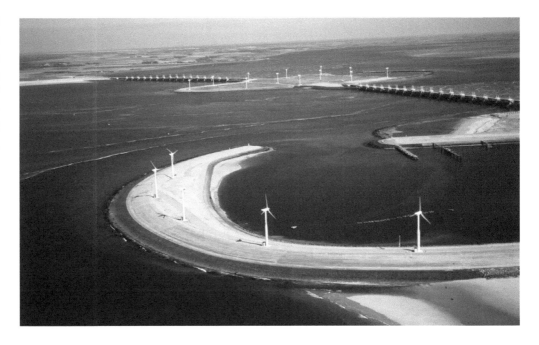

This flood barrier is part of Holland's Delta Project, a huge series of interconnecting dikes and barriers.

Project, began in 1958 and continued to 1997. The project includes 1,800 miles (3,000 kilometers) of dikes surrounding the country on the ocean side, and an additional series of 6,200 miles (10,000 kilometers) of dikes on inland canals and rivers. The Delta Project was one of the largest engineering tasks in history and is considered one of the seven wonders of the modern world. This series of dikes and dams is continually being strengthened and studied to prevent future vulnerabilities.

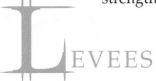

LEVEES

Levees are similar to dikes but are constructed to contain rivers rather than the sea. Simple levees are usually made from piles of dirt that are topped with sandbags or other material. To extend their capabilities, levees often take advantage of the natural terrain. For example, the riverside of a levee might be planted with Bermuda grass in order to help prevent erosion and keep the soil in place. Willow trees are sometimes planted, and artificial barriers, such as those made of concrete, are also used.

Levee systems are common in the Mississippi and Sacramento river deltas in the United States and are also found on rivers throughout

A road tops a levee that protects a low-elevation farm (top right) from the waters of the Sacramento River Delta in California.

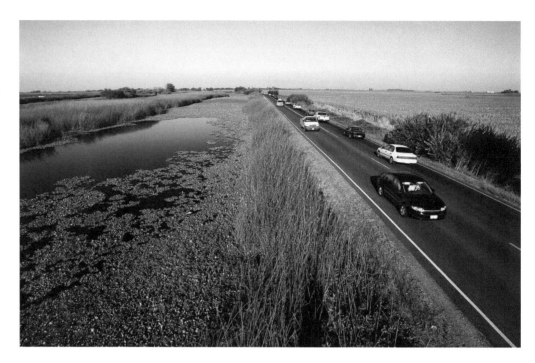

Europe. Levees were built in ancient times in regions where agriculture allowed large civilizations to develop along river valleys or in deltas and some basic flood control was required. Levees are found on Egypt's Nile River, in China, and in what was Mesopotamia, which lies in the Tigris-Euphrates valley.

Due to the physical properties of water, a levee system is only as strong as its weakest, or lowest, point. Water's equipotential surface spreads out into the lowest points of its channel or any other area available to it. If a river system is confined by a series of levees and the river level rises due to a flood or storm, the force of gravity will cause the water to break out of its confinement at the lowest point in the levee system.

It is useless to have walls that are 10 feet (3 meters) above the average water level in some places, if the walls are only 4 feet (1.2 meters) above the average water level in others. Storm or floodwater will break out of the channel at the location with the lowest wall height, or it will exploit other zones of weakness such as cracks or breaks in a levee. The development of a working levee system requires coordination and cooperation over a large land area, and historically it may have helped civilizations organize into larger cooperating societies.

Natural Levees

Levees occur naturally on most unconfined rivers that are allowed to meander freely. Rivers can either flow in their natural state or in a flood state. In a natural state, the river flows within the riverbanks and carries sediment with it downstream. When a river is in a flood state, as is the case seasonally in many parts of the world due to spring snow melt or monsoon rains, the river overflows its banks and spreads out over the floodplain. In spreading, the river's speed slows and the river can no longer carry as much suspended sediment in its water. The river deposits its sediment load in the floodplain, and the majority of the deposited material ends up on the banks of the river. This situation serves to build up natural levees along the sides of the river. In many places where a river is free from artificial or natural confinement, the banks of the river are built up by sediment deposits so that they are above the level of the surrounding floodplain.

Mississippi River Levees

The city of New Orleans, Louisiana, is situated between the Mississippi River and Lake Pontchartrain. As the area developed, swampland was drained to create more land for building. Similar to the situation in the Netherlands, draining the previous wetland caused the now-dry material to be compressed, and the ground level dropped. A complex series of levees was constructed to protect the city and its surrounding areas from potential flooding from the Mississippi River. The arrival of Hurricane Katrina in 2005, however, overtaxed this system and resulted in severe flooding and the complete evacuation of the city's residents.

The cause of the flooding of New Orleans is still under investigation. Hurricane Katrina was a huge, slow-moving storm with strong winds. The wind, waves, and rain from the storm resulted in an 18-foot (5.5-meter) rise in the amount of water in Lake Pontchartrain, located right next to New Orleans. Flood walls and levees began to collapse, and the city slowly flooded in the two days following the storm. Levees fail in one of two ways: either they are undermined and breached or they are overtopped. Undermining occurs when there is erosion at the base of a

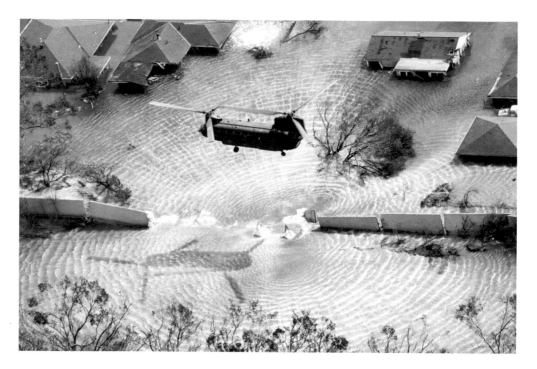

levee due to the pressure from large amounts of water or infiltration of storm water into the groundwater system directly below the levee. Overtopping means that water rises to a level that is higher than the height of a levee. Water washes over the top of the levee and can eventually wear a hole into the wall that is then exploited by more water.

It was originally thought that the levee failures following Hurricane Katrina were due to overtopping, but further investigation has suggested that the breaches were instead due to undermining. Investigators studying the soil underneath the New Orleans levees in the aftermath of

A levee is constructed from layers of permeable and nonpermeable materials. The river (left) applies a horizontal force to the base of the levee, which must be strong enough to withstand this pressure.

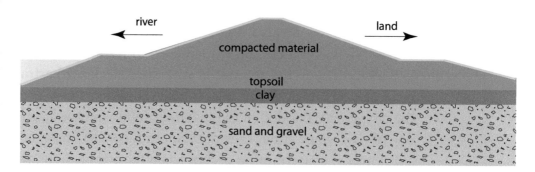

Hurricane Katrina found a thick layer of peat below the surface. This peat layer has a very low shear strength, which means that it can easily move in a horizontal direction; it also has a very high water content.

As the storm surge from Hurricane Katrina filled a canal lined by levees or flood walls, the water also infiltrated the soil and increased the water pressure in both the soil under the walls and the peat layer. Eventually, the water pressure reached a point where it was greater than the shear strength of the dirt and peat layer, and the entire layer suddenly shifted horizontally, taking the levee and its foundations with it. In one area, a section of the embankment of a levee that had supported a flood wall had moved 45 feet (18 meters) horizontally. If undermining of this sort was determined to have been the primary cause of the levee breaches, this would point to poor construction of the levees as a major cause of their failure. In areas where the levees remained intact, they were overtopped by the storm surge but were not breached, protecting those areas from serious flooding.

Seawalls

Seawalls protect both people and the natural environment against the powers of the ocean. These solid walls are built of a material like stone or concrete and are usually constructed parallel to the shoreline. Seawalls can also be built of materials such as wood or earth, but seawalls constructed this way tend to disintegrate over time and need to be replaced fairly often. Wooden and earthen seawalls are also more likely to be chewed away by local wildlife. Modern seawall building materials also include fiberglass and other polymers.

Reinforced concrete or large boulders are common choices for seawall construction because of their superior strength and weather-resistant properties. One disadvantage to a strong material like reinforced concrete, though, is that it essentially creates a dam. If water happens to pass over the top or around the sides of the seawall, it can remain trapped there and cause the soil underneath the seawall to erode, thereby lessening its strength and hastening its potential demise.

Seawalls are built to keep the ocean's waves from wearing away the natural shore. Water may seem benign, but over time it causes the erosion

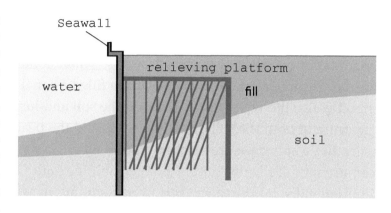

A seawall is a wall built right at the coastline to help spare the coast from further erosion. The water (left) applies a force to the seawall (right), which is filled in with dirt and supporting structures (middle).

of banks and other natural retaining devices. Supplementing a shoreline with a seawall helps to preserve the coastline.

Seawalls are generally vertical structures that are acted upon by a horizontal or angular force from the soil behind them. The seawall must be designed to support not only the weight of its materials but also this basal force. There is also the force of water hitting the seawall; this is a temporary load, but it must be considered in the planning of a seawall. These forces can be mitigated by designing a wall of sufficient width, in addition to providing a wider base for the seawall in cases where additional forces would warrant one. Seawalls need to withstand wildlife damage, saltwater corrosion, and major storm winds and waves.

While most seawalls are the silent heroes of the communities they serve, there have been a few exceptional cases where a seawall definitively saved a region from destruction. One such example is Pondicherry, a

FLOODGATES

Floodgates come in several different varieties. Radial gates have cylindrical walls that rotate to either allow water in or block it off. Bulkhead gates have large, movable, vertical walls that are raised or lowered depending on the need. Roller gates are typically cylindrical and can be rotated into open and closed positions.

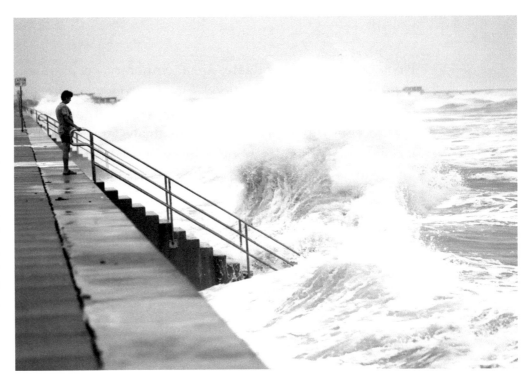

Seawalls, such as this one in Galveston, Texas, have helped protect the island city from many hurricanes. However, they were not high enough to block the devastation of Hurricane Ike, in 2008, which flooded much of the island.

city along the coast of India. A seawall was built in 1735, and it was made larger and stronger over the years. The current seawall is more than 1 mile (1.8 kilometers) long and averages around 25 feet (7.5 meters) high. In 2004, an earthquake measuring 9.0 on the Richter scale and centered in the Indian Ocean spawned a huge tsunami that went crashing to shore on India's coast. The strong stone seawall in Pondicherry probably saved the town from complete destruction.

Another life-saving seawall is found in Galveston, Texas. Galveston is located in a prime position to receive storms and winds from the Gulf of Mexico, and as the city's population grew over time, the potential damage from large storms grew as well. After a devastating hurricane killed thousands of people in 1900, the city commissioned the creation of a massive seawall 7 miles (11 kilometers) long in 1902. When the next major storm blew into town in 1918, the seawall did its job admirably, and fewer than ten people lost their lives. Over the years, the Galveston seawall was gradually extended. Today, the total length is nearly 10 miles (16 kilometers), the average height is about 17 feet (5 meters), and the base portions are as wide as 16 feet (4.8 meters).

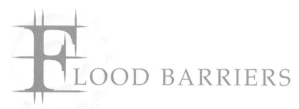

FLOOD BARRIERS

Flood barriers and floodgates are a temporary, yet at times critical, means of protecting a city from a flood. Flood barriers are movable walls that can be placed perpendicular to a river to keep it from flooding homes or other occupied portions of a city. Floodgates are adjustable doors that are usually installed under a bridge or on one side of a reservoir or river. They can be opened and closed as necessary to prevent a body of water from flowing too high.

A floodgate must withstand the force of the water acting against it. The amount of force acting on the floodgate can be calculated as a product of the pressure acting against it multiplied by the area of the gate:

$$F = PA$$

where F is the force, A is the area of the floodgate (width of the gate multiplied by the height of the submerged portion of the gate), and P is the pressure of the water pushing against the gate. This pressure can be calculated as:

$$P = \rho g h$$

where ρ is the density of fresh water, g is the acceleration from gravity, and h is the height of the water.

One of the world's most impressive flood barriers is called the Oosterscheldekering. It is located in the Netherlands and spans about 5.5 miles (9 kilometers). This was a large-scale project that took ten years to complete. It is part of a grouping of dams around the Netherlands built to protect the small country from storms and subsequent flooding. The project consists of a dam that rests on sixty-five pillars of concrete and a floodgate portion with massive steel gates.

Another giant flood barrier is the Thames River barrier, which protects the city of London from flooding. Six giant, rotating steel half-cylinders can be lowered to block the river if a dangerous surge tide approaches. The barriers block a stretch of the river that is 1,716 feet (523 meters) wide. The barrier became operational in 1982 and since then has been

TROPICAL DEPRESSION TWELVE

The devastation that occurred as a result of Hurricane Katrina originated not in Louisiana or Alabama, but in the Bahamas. Tropical Depression Twelve (what would later be known as Hurricane Katrina) was formed August 23, 2005, when a tropical wave came together with a tropical depression, or a closed system of thunderstorms and clouds. By August 24 the term "tropical storm" was applied to the burgeoning weather system; this means the high wind speeds defined it as a cyclone, and the name Katrina was bestowed at this time. Tropical Storm Katrina turned into Hurricane Katrina on August 25, when winds and rain became even more powerful.

Katrina first struck land in the southern part of Florida and temporarily weakened. It gained back its strength, and then some, while over the Gulf of Mexico. This additional power came from the hurricane's passing over the Loop Current, a deep ocean current warmer than other parts of the Gulf of Mexico. Warmer water fueled the hurricane, which then headed back toward land and resulted in the assault on Louisiana.

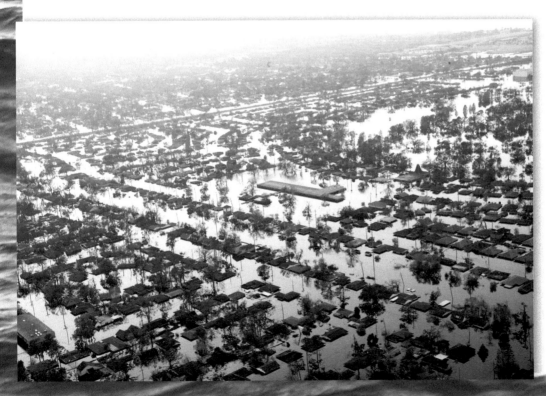

Hurricane Katrina breached the levees that protected the city of New Orleans, resulting in catastrophic flooding of much of the city.

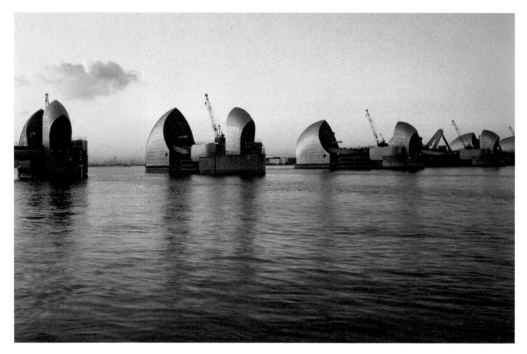

These gates, part of the Thames Barrier in England, can quickly block off the downstream portions of the river from an approaching flood.

used almost 100 times in response to flood conditions. The barrier was built to compensate for predicted rising sea levels until at least 2030. If sea levels continue to rise at the same rate as they are today, a larger barrier will need to be put in place by then.

A similar flood barrier was proposed in the 1960s to protect the city of New Orleans from hurricanes. Construction of this barrier began in 1971, but it was halted due to lawsuits over its predicted environmental impact. After years of court battles, the U.S. Army Corps of Engineers decided to reinforce the levee system instead. In the wake of Hurricane Katrina, it is unclear if this was the right decision.

While water is the lifeblood of humanity, it can also be one of mankind's greatest threats. Rivers and other water sources are vital to civilization, but they must be properly harnessed in order for people to take advantage of the water without its becoming a danger. Fortunately, many effective means of water management have been developed over the years and are employed in different manifestations worldwide. From dams and levees to waterwheels and canals, the design of dams and waterways is a fascinating study.

GLOSSARY

Activation energy—the threshold energy that must be overcome in order for some other action to take place

Aqueduct—a structure that transports water from one place to another

Aquifer—a layer of underground rock that is saturated with water

Arable land—land that can be used for farming

Arch dams—thin curved dams that are similar to arch bridges and use their shape to resist the forces of water they must support

Arid—having insufficient rainfall to support agriculture

Atom—the smallest particle of any element that contains all of that element's properties

Bevel gears—gears that fit together at a right angle and therefore change the resulting direction of rotation

Buoyancy—the upward force exerted on a body in water that causes the object to float rather than sink

Buttress dam—type of dam that has a smooth wall on the upstream side and a series of braced supports on the downstream side

Calving—the process of a small iceberg breaking off from a larger one

Canal—a man-made, or artificial, water passage

Canal lock—a physical construction that helps lift a boat between changes in water level of a canal

Cistern—a container for storing water or other liquids

Cyclone—a storm caused by a low-pressure area with winds that typically blow counterclockwise

Dike—a long embankment that protects against flooding from a body of water

Electromagnetic induction—the creation of an induced electric field through the motion of a conductor through a magnetic field; discovered by Michael Faraday in 1831; used for power generation in hydroelectric power plants

Embankment dams—huge sloped piles of dirt and rubble, with a waterproof central core, that do not allow water to seep through

Equipotential surface—a surface that forms to lie at a constant value of gravitational potential energy; for example, water will form an equipotential surface in which the water is approximately the same absolute distance from the center of the Earth in all places, such as at sea level

Evaporation—a phase change whereby, for example, water changes from a liquid to a gas

Flash lock—a device such as a door or gate in the middle of a dam wall or weir

Flood barrier—movable wall that can be placed perpendicular to a river in order to keep it from flooding homes or other occupied portions of a city

Floodplain—low-lying terrain that may be subject to flooding

Floodgate—adjustable door that is usually installed under a bridge or on one side of a reservoir or river

Friction—the force of resistance encountered by touching objects as they move past each other

Gear ratio—the distance between the center of a gear and the place where the gear contacts another object

Gravitational potential energy—a type of potential energy in which the stored energy is increased by virtue of its elevated position

Gravity dams—massive concrete dams that hold up to the forces of water pressure simply through their huge mass

Gristmill—a mill for grinding grain

Hydroelectric power—electricity generated from water

Infiltration—the movement of water from the surface into underlying soil

Irrigation—supplying water by constructed or artificial means

Irrigation canal—a long man-made ditch that diverts water from a nearby river or lake to where it is needed to water crops

Kinetic energy—the energy of a body in motion

Levee—an embankment that runs parallel to a river or other body of water

Molecule—the smallest unit of any substance that contains all of that substance's properties; composed of more than one atom

Navigation lock—a chamber that allows boats to travel a canal in places where the water level changes, usually due to the surrounding terrain

Overshot waterwheel—a type of waterwheel that works by gravity; water falls from an aqueduct or waterfall above the wheel, forcing the wheel to turn

Overtopping—a condition that occurs when storm or floodwaters rise to a level that is higher than the height of the dikes or levees meant to contain them

Potential energy—the stored energy held by a body

Precipitation—water falling to the earth (rain, snow, sleet, etc.)

Pumped storage plant—a type of hydroelectric power plant that contains two separate reservoirs, one located at a high elevation and one lower

River engineering—the science of willfully diverting or otherwise influencing the course of a river, usually to provide humans with a particular benefit

Sawmill—a building in which lumber is taken and cut down to size for use in construction or other applications

Seawall—a solid wall, built of a material like stone or concrete, usually constructed parallel to the shore to protect the land from erosion

Sediment—particles such as soil and sand that tend to sink to the bottom of rivers, streams, lakes, and other bodies of water

Shaft—a bar that extends out perpendicularly from a wheel's center when used as part of an assembly

Shear strength—the ability of a material, such as soil, to withstand shear forces

Shear stress—a state created by parallel planes sliding against each other

Silt—small particles of sediment

Sinkhole—a hole in the ground that occurs when a layer of rock is dissolved by naturally occurring groundwater

Siphon—a tube or structure used to carry water from a higher to a lower elevation

Surface tension—the attractive force of molecules on water's surface

Temperate—describes a climate with a moderate temperature

Triple point of water—the point at which water can exist in all three phases (solid, liquid, and gas) at the same time

Tropical depression—a cyclone with relatively low wind speeds

Typhoon—hurricanes that originate in the North Pacific or the China Sea, with wind speeds of greater than 74 mph (120 km/h)

Undermining—a condition that results when erosion occurs at the base of a levee

Undershot waterwheel—a type of waterwheel that is generally located in a stream or river; the forceful flow of the water turns the wheel

Water cycle—a description of how Earth's water moves between the three phases of solid, liquid, and gas, as well as the physical movement of water over the surface

Water table—the point where water in the ground is stable, coinciding with the physical level at which the soil is saturated with water

Weir—a low overflow dam that raises the water level in part of a canal

FIND OUT MORE

Books

American Water Works Association. *Water Treatment Plant Design.* Columbus, OH: McGraw-Hill, 2004.

Barry, John. *Rising Tide: The Great Mississippi Flood of 1927 and How It Changed America.* New York: Simon and Schuster, 1998.

Baker, Lindsay. *A Field Guide to American Windmills.* Norman: University of Oklahoma Press, 1985.

Hecht, Roger. *The Erie Canal Reader.* Syracuse, NY: Syracuse University Press, 2003.

Koeppel, Gerard. *Water for Gotham: A History.* Princeton, NJ: Princeton University Press, 2001.

McDonald, Dylan. *The Teton Dam Disaster.* San Francisco: Arcadia, 2006.

Priwer, Shana, and Cynthia Phillips. *The Everything Da Vinci Book.* Cincinnati, OH: Adams Media, 2006.

Van Heerden, Ivor. *The Storm: What Went Wrong and Why During Hurricane Katrina.* New York: Viking, 2006.

Varble, Derek. *The Suez Crisis, 1956.* Westminster: Osprey, 2003.

Verma, Balraj. *The Beautiful India: Pondicherry.* Ontario: Reference Press, 2006.

Web sites

Beaver Dam Information Site: www.beaverdam.info

Dealing with the Deluge: www.pbs.org/wgbh/nova/flood/deluge.html

Galveston Historical Foundation: www.galvestonhistory.org

National Renewable Energy Laboratory: www.nrel.gov

Nova Secrets of Lost Empires: Roman Baths:
    www.pbs.org/wgbh/nova/lostempires/roman

The Panama Canal Authority: www.pancanal.com

Science Daily: Anthropologist Examines the Power of Water on Earth's
    Earliest Civilizations:
    www.sciencedaily.com/releases/2001/02/010221071726.htm

The Water Cycle: http://ga.water.usgs.gov/edu/watercycle.html

Water History: www.waterhistory.org

Water Properties: http://ga.water.usgs.gov/edu/waterproperties.html

World Atlas of Maps, Flags and Geography Facts and Figures:
    http://worldatlas.com

INDEX

Page numbers in italics refer to illustrations.